"By compiling and editing this superb volume, David Scharff has made an important contribution to our field. Each of the original and informative essays in the book enhances our understanding and appreciation of the various uses of the object, a topic of great importance and one that has been much neglected in the literature. This landmark work not only corrects that deficiency, but provides a valuable educational experience for students and practitioners alike. This is a book that belongs in the library of every analytic therapist."

—**Theodore Jacobs**, MD, member of the New York Psychoanalytic Association, Author, *The Use of the Self* and *The Possible Profession.*

"This highly original book hugely extends the study of the variety of ways in which we may use our objects, and for that matter, misuse them or be misused by them. Disturbing interactions between internal and powerful external objects are examined, and careful distinctions between oedipal and pre-oedipal matters always carefully observed. There is deep and moving analytic work and thinking being carried out here. Prepare to be edified and surprised!"

—**Anne Alvarez**, PhD, MACP. Consultant Child and Adolescent Psychotherapist. Author, *Live Company* and *The Thinking Heart.*

The Use of the Object in Psychoanalysis

Using Winnicott's classic paper as its starting point, this fascinating collection explores a range of clinical and theoretical psychoanalytic perspectives around relating to "the object." Each author approaches the topic from a different angle, switching among the patient's use of others in their internal and external lives, their use of their therapist, and the therapist's own use of their patients.

The use of objects is susceptible to wide interpretation and elaboration; it is both a normal phenomenon and a marker for certain personal difficulties, or even psychopathologies, seen in clinical practice. While it is normal for people to relate to others through the lens of their internal objects in ways that give added meaning to aspects of their lives, it becomes problematic when people live as if devoid of a self and instead live almost exclusively through the others who form their internal worlds, often leading them to feel that they cannot be happy until and unless others change.

Assessing the significance of objects among adult and child patients, groups and the group-as-object, and exploring Freud's own use of objects, *The Use of the Object in Psychoanalysis* will be of significant interest both to experienced psychoanalysts and psychotherapists and to trainees exploring important theoretical questions.

David E. Scharff, MD, is Co-Founder and Chair Emeritus of the Board, International Psychotherapy Institute, Chair of the International Psychoanalytic Association's Committee on Couple and Family Psychoanalysis, and Editor of the journal *Psychoanalysis and Psychotherapy in China.*

The Use of the Object in Psychoanalysis

An Object Relations Perspective on the Other

Edited by David E. Scharff

Routledge
Taylor & Francis Group
LONDON AND NEW YORK

First published 2020
by Routledge
2 Park Square, Milton Park, Abingdon, Oxon OX14 4RN

and by Routledge
52 Vanderbilt Avenue, New York, NY 10017

Routledge is an imprint of the Taylor & Francis Group, an informa business

British Library Cataloguing-in-Publication Data
A catalogue record for this book is available from the British Library

Library of Congress Cataloging-in-Publication Data
A catalog record for this book has been requested

ISBN: 978-0-367-18915-0 (hbk)
ISBN: 978-0-367-18916-7 (pbk)
ISBN: 978-0-429-19917-2 (ebk)

Typeset in Times
by Apex CoVantage, LLC

Contents

Contributors

Ron B. Aviram, PhD, is an Adjunct Associate Professor at Ferkauf Graduate School of Psychology at Yeshiva University. He is author of *The Relational Origins of Prejudice: A convergence of psychoanalytic and social cognitive psychology*. He is in private practice in New York City. ronaviram@msn.com

Carl Bagnini, LCSW, BCD, is founding and senior faculty, The International Psychotherapy Institute; Faculty, The Gordon Derner Post-Graduate Psychoanalytic Institute and The Training Institute for Mental Health. Author, *Keeping Couples in Treatment – Working from Surface to Depth*, and is in private practice in Port Washington, NY. edre54@aol.com

Nancy L. Bakalar, MD, is a graduate of The International Institute for Psychoanalysis (IIPT), where she is a supervising analyst and teaching faculty member. She is also a faculty member of The Denver Institute for Psychoanalysis. She developed and taught in the Infant Observation Program at The International Psychotherapy Institute (IPI) for ten years. She is a Distinguished Fellow of the American Psychiatric Association and practices psychoanalysis and individual, couple, and family psychodynamic psychotherapy in person and by videoteleconference in a suburb of Denver, Colorado. nlbakalar@comcast.net

James L. Poulton, PhD, is a psychologist in private practice in Salt Lake City, Utah, an Adjunct Assistant Professor in Psychology at the University of Utah, and a member of the national faculty of the International Psychotherapy Institute. He has written numerous articles and chapters on psychoanalytic theory and treatment and is the author of *Object Relations and Relationality in Couple Therapy: Exploring the Middle Ground* and co-author of *Internalization: The Origin and Construction of Internal Reality*. jlpoulton@mac.com

David E. Scharff, MD, is Emeritus Chair of the Board, Co-Founder, and Former Director, International Psychotherapy Institute; Chair, The International Psychoanalytic Association's Committee on Family and Couple Psychoanalysis; Clinical Professor of Psychiatry, Uniformed Services University of the Health Sciences and Georgetown University; Supervising Analyst, International Institute for Psychoanalytic Training; Teaching Analyst, Washington Psychoanalytic Institute; Honorary Fellow, Tavistock Relationships, London;

Former President, American Association of Sex Educators, Counselors and Therapists, and former Vice President, International Association for Couple and Family Psychoanalysis. He is a child and adult analyst in private practice with children, adults, couples, and families in Chevy Chase, Maryland. He is the author and editor of more than 30 books, with foundational texts on family, couple, and individual psychoanalytic therapy, the work of Ronald Fairbairn and of Enrique Pichon Rivière, sexual difficulty, and innovative training of psychotherapists and psychoanalysts. His recent initiatives involve organizing training programs in Russia and in China, where he has founded an innovative training program for students from across China. To this end he is founder of a journal devoted to the newly emergent field of psychoanalysis in China, called *Psychoanalysis and Psychotherapy in China*. As Chair of the Couple and Family Psychoanalysis Committee of the International Psychoanalytic Association, he has, together with members of the group, organized meetings of the committee and international congresses that further the study of family and couple psychoanalysis around the world. davidscharff@theipi.org

Jill Savege Scharff is an internationally known psychoanalyst for children and adults, couples and families. She is the co-founder and former co-director of the International Psychotherapy Institute. She was the founding Chair of the International Institute for Psychoanalytic Training, the analytic training program at the International Psychotherapy Institute, where she also developed an analytic supervision training program, a child therapy and child analytic curriculum. She is a teaching analyst at the Washington Center for Psychoanalysis and a clinical professor of psychiatry at Georgetown University. Her private practice is in Chevy Chase, Maryland. She is the author of *Projective and Introjective Identification and the Use of the Therapist's Self* (1992) and senior co-author with David E. Scharff of *The Primer of Object Relations: Second Edition* (2005), *Tuning the Therapeutic Instrument: Affective Learning of Psychotherapy* (2000), *Object Relations Individual Therapy* (1998), and *Object Relations Therapy of Physical and Sexual Trauma* (1996). With David E. Scharff as the senior author, Jill Savege Scharff co-wrote many books on object relations: *Object Relations Family Therapy* (1987), *Object Relations Couple Therapy* (1991), *and The Interpersonal Unconscious* (2012). She is co-series editor with David E. Scharff of the Library of Object Relations at Jason Aronson (now at Rowman and Littlefield) and series editor of the Library of Technology and Mental Health at Routledge. She has edited four books in the *Psychoanalysis Online* series (Routledge, 2013, 2015, 2017, and 2019). jillscharff@theipi.org

Caroline Sehon, MD, FABP, Chair and Supervising Analyst, International institute for Psychoanalytic Training (IIPT) at the International Psychotherapy Institute (IPI); Teaching and Supervising Faculty in IPI's child and adult psychotherapy training programs; Clinical Associate Professor of Psychiatry at Georgetown University. Adult and child psychoanalyst and psychiatrist in private practice in Bethesda, Maryland. Author of papers and chapters on object relations individual, couple and family therapy. carolinesehon@gmail.com

Juan Tubert-Oklander, MD, PhD, is a psychoanalyst and group analyst, living and practicing in Mexico City. Full Member of the Argentine Psychoanalytic Association and the International Psychoanalytical Association, Honorary Member of the Group-Analytic Society International, Founding Member of the International Field Theory Association, and Member of the International Association of Relational Psychoanalysis and Psychotherapy. Professor in the Master´s Degree Course of Psychoanalytic Psychotherapy at the Marista University of Merida. Author of numerous papers and book chapters, published in Spanish, English, Italian, French, Portuguese, Czech, and Hebrew. Co-author, with Reyna Hernández-Tubert, of *Operative Groups: The Latin-American Approach to Group Analysis* (Jessica Kingsley, 2004) and author of *Theory of Psychoanalytical Practice: A Relational Process Approach* (IPA/Karnac, 2013) and *The One and the Many: Relational Psychoanalysis and Group Analysis* (London: Karnac, 2014), as well as several books in Spanish. jtubertoklander@gmail.com

Introduction

How do we use others?

David E. Scharff

The question of how we relate to important people in our lives is a different question from how we use them. Winnicott wrote that object relating preceded object using – a statement that seemed so counterintuitive to me that I have puzzled over it on and off for the many years since I first read *Playing and Reality* soon after it was published.

I did not meet Winnicott, although I had planned a year's sabbatical in London partially with the hope of learning directly from him and from John Bowlby. Winnicott had died at a relatively early an age not long before I arrived. Nevertheless, there were others interested in his work who had known him well and with whom I was able to interact, allowing me to learn from them. There was the whole world of British psychoanalysis – Klein, Fairbairn, Bowlby, and Bion – to reckon with. Of the group, Bowlby was in the middle of writing his landmark three-volume study, *Attachment and Loss*, and very present at the Tavistock Clinic. There were enigmas embedded in the work of each. Fairbairn and Bowlby seemed the most logical and coherent; Klein, passionate but difficult to muddle through. Bion was not yet in the forefront of my London teachers' minds but became more so when he returned to London from California and taught them directly a few years later. So, later, I was able to learn from those whom he had mentored himself when they came to Washington, DC, to work with my colleagues and me.

There are other notable schools of thought about how we use others. In the United States, the intersubjective and relational schools have contributed greatly to our ideas about shared unconscious processes, and in South America, from Pichon-Rivière on and including the work of such eminent analysts as Jose Bleger, Isidoro Berenstein, Janine Puget, and Julio Moreno, with elaboration in Europe by Rene Kaës and Antonino Ferro, ideas of the interactive links (or *el vinculo*) between people have recently come to feature more prominently in the English-language analytic dialogue.

In the United States, I have had the particular pleasure of learning from Theodore Jacobs, whose landmark articles and presentations, published in his book *The Use of the Object*, have explored the ways countertransference and all subjective experience with patients informs our work. I conceived the idea for this book while thinking of his work. I think of "the use of the object" as a counterpoint to

Jacobs's conception of "the use of the self," although, of course, the two concepts overlap and intermingle greatly.

Each of these theorist/clinicians has informed me, occupied a part of my mind, for considerable periods. In this way, each has been an object whom I have used ruthlessly, if with a large measure of awe for what they were able to discover and formulate. But there are continuing ways that I and many of us keep coming back to Winnicott and his enigmatic way of thinking that so often leads to a depth of exploration.

This book is a series of essays formed around the attempt to explore and intuit "uses of the object." Precisely because this theme is susceptible to wide interpretation and elaboration, each essay starts from the author's personal and sometimes idiosyncratic take on the question.

From the beginning, I realized that the question of the use of the object – and the larger theme of uses of others – is subject to multiple explorations and multiple meanings. While I had a rough idea of what I had in mind even before writing my own chapter, I knew that no one essay could exhaust the vectors that could be usefully applied to looking at how people use both their external objects or the people in their lives or how they relate to the internal objects that are part of their own psychic structure. I realized that using objects was both a normal phenomenon and marker for a particular kind of personal difficulty or even psychopathology that I experience in clinical practice. It is normal for people to have internal objects whom they treasure and who give a kind of meaning to aspects of their life that they would not otherwise experience. But it becomes problematic when people live almost exclusively through the others who form their internal world, then often coming to feel that they cannot be happy until and unless their others change. In the clinical situation, they often come with the aim of changing the other person, whether they say so directly or only behave as though this is their goal without saying so.

Having formulated this problem, I then went about enlisting colleagues who I thought would be particularly interested in and qualified to explore this area with me. Ultimately, this formed the basis of a year-long series of seminars and led to fruitful exchange. The chapters in this book come directly from those presentations and discussions, rewritten in the light of the discussions among our group of colleagues.

In Chapter 1, I discuss patients who taught me about this concept, ending with a patient whose growth allowed her to begin to surrender the organization of living in and through her bad objects. In Chapter 2, James L. Poulton asks the fundamental question of psychic organization, "What does the other have to do with our inner lives?" Chapter 3, by Carl Bagnini, explores the often painful process of dreaming our internal objects during therapy, finding them again, and grieving for lost objects. Caroline Sehon explores shadows of inner object worlds in Chapter 4, and Nancy L. Bakalar looks at an analysis through the long lens of "The analyst's self as object for the patient" in Chapter 5. Chapters 6 and 7 are each different in focus from the ones that have come before. In Chapter 6, Ron B. Aviram explores a concept he has described as the "social object," a group object that inhabits us. Juan Tubert-Oklander's Chapter 7 is the most theoretical, as he traces the history of analytic ideas about humankind's social nature. Finally, Jill Savege Scharff's concluding Chapter 8 is the most personal. Her discussion ranges from her own experience with patients to the fact that she, as both my colleague and my wife, is writing such a chapter that explores the ultimately personal issue of the internal object in self and other.

From all these perspectives, it is my hope that this volume of explorations will open a previously neglected area for analytic discourse. In this way, living with and often in our analytic objects – as all analytic therapists do – we can use them in a benign and growth-promoting way in order to come to understand our work and ourselves anew.

1 Living in the object

David E. Scharff

To discuss patients who live their emotional lives by what I have come to call "living in the objects," I began by re-reading Winnicott's (1971) article from *Playing and Reality*, "The use of an object and relating through identifications." This is not an easy article, because what he says is that *object relating* comes first and begins when the infant is in a merged state with the mother. Then it is through the destruction of the object and yet having the object survive that destructive set of acts toward the object that the other person becomes real for the infant. It then becomes possible for the infant to use the object in a set of real relationships between two subjects. In this way, Winnicott puts destruction at the center of the growth of a capacity to form emotional relationships between two people, each of whom has his or her own autonomous inner lives and who then relate to each other across what he defined a *potential or transitional space* through the use of *transitional phenomena.*

Destruction of the merged object is therefore at the center of his postulation of a developmental sequence toward mutual relating. This growth in capacity to use the object is at the center of a maturational line that has to do with the capacity to relate to somebody else with what Winnicott called a *capacity for concern*, his language for Melanie Klein's depressive position.

In thinking about the idea of "the use of the object," I realized that I had something else in mind, an elaboration of one part of Winnicott's paradigm. I want to explore the way in which our patients, and people in general, use the idea of another person for their own purposes. Of course, everybody does this in health and illness, but some of our patients come to us through the particular mental mechanism of *using the image of another person as a long-term substitute for a sense of having an inner life of their own.*

This idea came to me many years ago through experience with a patient who I came to feel *had a sense of being alive only when talking about his wife.* His wife was a wealthy woman, whose wealth was inherited and not the fruit of her own work or of his, and who lived in a world of excess. She shopped tirelessly and spent excessively. She used the sense of whether he was willing to indulge her, as her father had indulged her before him, as the sign of whether he loved her and obeyed her – or not.

Notice that I have introduced this man mainly by talking about his wife. I'll call him Mikey because that's like the kind of infantilizing name by which the family called him. Talking about his wife is exactly what he did. He talked only about his wife. It was the damnedest thing. I could not get him to talk about himself except through focusing on what his wife wanted of him and the travails she exposed him to. He explained to me, actually he complained to me, that she would buy things, get tired of them, and ask him to resell them for her, usually at some fraction of the original cost. Nevertheless, although he could sell them only for, let's say, half of what they originally cost, the income from these resales was substantial enough that it was crucial to supporting their current lifestyle, which was otherwise constrained by what the family trust money would allow them. Mikey was exasperated by her getting and spending, her selling and spending again. He talked about it all the time. He would have to arrange to return or resell the things, call the stores to manage their credit points (on which they also relied for buying yet more things), and attempt to rein her in because his mother-in-law was constantly on him to manage his wife's overspending. And he had to manage the family business for the whole coterie of the three daughters and a slightly no-account son, a business inherited from his deceased father-in-law and on which they were all dependent.

Mikey's wife was in therapy, too, but she complained that the therapy put uncomfortable pressure on her to examine her life. Because we had permission to speak, her therapist was able to confirm to me that Mikey's description of his wife's life and her constant complaints about any constraints he put on her was pretty much the way Mikey described it. Although my understanding was that her therapist worked hard about putting even gentle pressure on her toward self-examination, just the pressure of being in therapy and the invitation to look into her own behavior and way of living at all was more than she could stand. Soon she chafed at the prospect of continuing therapy and then began to feel that my work with Mikey threatened to unravel his compliance with her wishes. She began to lobby him to stop therapy. Mikey said to me, "I like coming here. I feel you are the only person I can talk to about the life I lead. But I'm going to have to stop because, if I don't, everything in my life will fall apart." So, he complied with his wife's pressure and stopped.

In the middle of treating Mikey, it had occurred to me that, inside his mind, he had no independent life. His only way of feeling alive was to be inside his wife. His inner object of her served as substitute for an inner sense of self. Metaphorically, and unconsciously, he *lived inside his wife*. I formulated this to myself: that "he lived in his object." It was as though he had no life outside his thoughts about her.

My formulation of Mikey's problem also stemmed from my countertransference. Gradually, I came to realize that when I was with him, I would be longing for him to "get a life" outside his complaints about his wife. That was my crude formulation of a longing for him to develop a self, to develop a masculine capacity to confront her and actually to confront himself. My countertransference was my early guide to the specifics of what seemed to be missing in his inner world.

Once I had formulated the idea for myself that Mikey lived in his object, I realized that to a certain extent everybody does this. The people who are important to us define who we are. Our struggles with them are the struggles of ourselves in action, in relationship to the most important people in our lives. To a large extent, we all live through our objects.

How different is this dyadic formulation from an Oedipal version of the same problem? A three-year-old girl who had quite a lovely relationship with her mother said to her, “You’re a bad mommy.” “Who isn’t bad?” asked her mother. “Daddy is a good daddy!” the girl said. From having a previously good overall relationship with her mother, she was facing her developmental challenge by formulating the Oedipal version of inhabiting a bad object, splitting it off from the idealized object. We all know this psychic formula, but my point here is that this leads to a familiar pattern of patients (and other people) who live in this formulation, who cannot forgive their mothers or fathers, and who live in and through grievances with or idealizations of them.

This is a very different from the way Winnicott formulated the situation. For him, object relating came first. He dated the capacity for creative destruction of the object, with the aim of being able to create a new object, as the beginning of mutuality. It is in this paper that he states that the object was there before the infant created it, but the mother must not challenge the infant’s sense that the infant created the new object. It is the creative act, founded in creative destructiveness, that opens a place for discovery of the real world of relationships. Mikey would have had to be able to destroy the image of his self-centered wife as all-powerful and displacing all room for him to have an independently operating mind. He could not bear to carry out that act of destruction. It was not her refusal to allow him independence that was the problem – although she certainly did forbid it. It was his own act of *forbidding himself* to challenge her and risk losing her in the attempt to spur her growth and his own. That he could not face.

In the ordinary process of development, we hope that our children will destroy the image of us as all-powerful and as constituting their sole universe, so that they can develop new relationships with each of us as they grow up and so they can develop the capacity to relate to others with mutual give-and-take. We hope they will not simply live inside these other people as their inner objects.

So, what is the process of doing this in a way that is beyond the enigma of Winnicott’s description? And, in a parallel way, what is the pathology of failure to accomplish this developmental task?

Thinking through this line becomes easier once we include the conception of the link as formulated by Pichon-Rivière (Scharff, Losso and Setton, 2017; Losso, de Setton and Scharff, 2017). Conceptually the link is formed as an external structure in the space between two people or between members of a group. Its organization is developed by these people interacting, and, in turn, it organizes the individuals themselves who make up the link. A link is an interactional structure formed by a combination of individuals’ unconscious and conscious interactions, the movements of their bodies and their speech. It represents an organization in the space between the people and between their minds; that is, the totality of their interacting relationship. Then, in turn, this link pattern contributes to their continuing re-organization.

Then the link itself is represented in the mind of each of the individuals. Pichon-Rivière followed Fairbairn's description of the psyche as formed by a series of self-and-object links (1952). These internal linked organizations are themselves in constant dynamic interaction inside the mind. The organization of mind is a fractal of the external link between emotional partners. The minds of each partner are constantly reformed by their dynamic link, and they constantly contribute to ongoing links with the social world.

Therefore, when we talk about somebody living in the object, we are describing a person who lives psychically at one pole of a bipolar internal organization. In ordinary life, people live with an oscillation between aspects of their organized self and aspects of their internal object organizations. Internal objects are, as Fairbairn described, parts of the mind. Both self and object are parts of the ego capable of generating activity. Our internal objects can be the organizers through which we speak, just as our self-organizations are.

For instance, an adolescent patient berates her therapist. On examination it turns out that she is treating the therapist the way she feels her mother treats her. At this moment in therapy, it is irrelevant whether the mother actually treats her so badly or whether this is a construction she makes of a mother who is simply setting limits. While we understand that such a teenager is more likely to feel that she has an actually cruel mother and that the degree of cruelty will feel worse if mother is actually behaving cruelly to her, at the moment in the therapy that is not the point. The point at that moment is that our teenage patient is speaking from her internal object rather than from the aspect of herself, who, in this exchange, feels mistreated. Instead, it is the therapist in her countertransference who feels mistreated just now. At other times such an adolescent speaks for herself, complaining about how she suffers at the hands of her mother or, even on a good day, saying, "My mother's not really so bad, but sometimes she just gives me a pain." That is to say, a patient who is relatively healthy is capable of speaking from her self-organization and less often speaks from the sense that she is living inside the bad internal object. Of course, an internal object can also be good-enough. In this position, the girl would be saying kind things about a world that otherwise she might be inclined to speak ill of. Or the internal object can be idealized, as when somebody speaks from the position of living in the idealized or exciting internal object, as happens in the passion of young romance.

So, it seems to me that Mikey was embodying a particular kind of pathology of the use of an object. He was *living in* his indispensable bad object. His is the pathology of someone who is trapped in the world of his internal object, with no perspective other than that of the internal object or, at least, no perspective other than the focus on and sense of living inside a constraining relationship with that internal object. There is no feeling of mutuality in this sense of being trapped. Unconsciously, such patients are organized by the sense that "I need to do something either to be obedient to the internal object or to be constantly in a battle with it because it defines who I am, who I am allowed to be." This sense is unconscious, although there are always important conscious derivatives of it. That is, one can be entirely conscious of a feeling that the world is dominated by this figure. From our perspective, it is an internal object, but to the person the other is a constant presence in his or her mind that determines almost everything that the person does or feels – mood, organization, and orientation toward the world. But the reasons for living this way psychically are centered in the person's sense of being trapped and are principally unconscious fantasies. More important, these are unconscious axioms about how the person must live. Therefore, such patients are often rather unavailable to therapists, as these axioms are held to be unquestioned truths about the only way they can relate to the important people in their lives. If there are people in these patients' lives who would like to have a more mutual relationship, that mutuality has to be denied.

Here is an example that will be familiar to child and family therapists.

Quentin came to me because his wife, Samantha, could not let go of the idea that her 14-year-old son, Adam, was up to no good in one way or another. She worried incessantly about Adam and could not let go of her preoccupation with him. According to Quentin's description, she was living in her son-as-object. This man thought that his son was doing fine. "He's a little laconic, it's true. He doesn't seem to have any great ambitions, but he has cottoned on to the art program at school with great enthusiasm. And he generally gets As, with the exception of history, which he doesn't like but in which he still gets a B. It's true he spends a lot of time in his room, that he wanders around the neighborhood with a changing combination of friends, and that we don't really know who the friends are." This preoccupation of Samantha's meant that there was a great deal of strain in the couple's relationship, too, since Quentin got along better with Adam than with his wife, sharing activities like tennis, which occasionally he and his son played together. Adam actually did seem to work on his tennis fairly actively. He refused to take lessons but had taught himself fairly well.

We could say that this man was partly living in the middle of his wife's distress, living in her as an object. Certainly, he presented the situation as constraining his relationship with her, and that is the problem he brought to me. He presented this as more of a problem than the fact that he drank more than she wished and that drinking had been a constant factor in the evenings at home. He traveled a great deal for work, something he no longer enjoyed, and he felt pretty washed out when he got home from a job that had become a burden. However, what distinguishes Quentin from the example of Mikey is that Quentin had another life in the sense that he talked about other relationships – his life at work, his own aspirations and interests. So, he was living in his internal constrained object only to the extent that this was a problem in his life.

Later on, Samantha became obsessed with the idea that Adam was on drugs. As a result, she searched his room and his backpack and found a small vial of a powdery substance. They sent it for testing, and it turned out it was a synthetic of marijuana. This confirmed her darkest suspicions, while for the husband this was the kind of ordinary problem that parents face these days, something to be taken seriously but not a calamity. What Quentin regretted most was the fear that this confirmation of his wife's preoccupation not just would become the defining element of her relationship with her son, which was impaired by her suspicions of him, but also would also come to totally define Quentin's relationship with his wife.

This woman was *living in* the worrisome object of her son, a part of herself that she was terribly worried about as going bad, being out of control and going down a path of destruction. And her living in the worrisome object-son then affected her marital relationship so that her husband was living in her – or, perhaps more accurately, in the worrisome mother-son pair as a combined inner object – in a parallel preoccupation. (I did have confirmation of this formulation about her from Samantha's therapist since we were authorized to talk.)

I suggested that we have a family session. Adam had refused to have treatment earlier when he had been so apparently lacking in motivation, but now, with this discovery, Quentin was able to make the case that Adam no longer had a choice. In the session Quentin and Samantha were able to confront Adam about what he had done. He understood that he had been caught red-handed. Taking advantage of this crisis in their family, we were able to discuss Adam's feeling that his mother did not trust him and that this distrust colored their entire relationship.

When I asked Samantha about the possible origins of her fear about Adam, she connected it to her schizophrenic brother. In his late teen years, he had suddenly become psychotic. He had never recovered, never been able to have a productive life. She had spent her life after her parents' death taking care of him. She connected her preoccupation with Adam with her constant fear. She was afraid that there might be some sign that she would miss that Adam would come to the same fate, and so any hint of a misstep on his part brought out her tremendous fears for his development. In the session, she was able to say that she felt he communicated so little to her about his life that the gap between them fueled her fear and suspiciousness, while admitting that her position of being suspicious of him all the time amounted to what Samantha called a "paranoid position." She owned up to the idea that she carried this preoccupation in excess of anything that he had done to provoke it, and that this had informed a malignant element in their relationship. She said to Adam, "But If you would only talk to me more, just to tell me ordinary things about your life, it would help me in my own attempts to control this so it would not contaminate our relationship."

Adam said that he wanted more freedom than he had in the past, because he was getting older and he thought he behaved generally in a responsible way. He maintained the story that this synthetic marijuana was put in his backpack by a friend and that he had nothing to do with it, but he agreed that its discovery justified his parents' suspiciousness. Nevertheless, he said, he would like more sense of trust from them, more independence, although he still wanted to be connected to them. In his turn, Quentin was able to say to his wife that her unrelenting suspiciousness about their son had a negative impact on their relationship, too. He wanted a return of the sense of freedom from constraint that had characterized their early relationship. He experienced her having a child as something that provoked her worries in a way that impinged on the sense of a more loving mutuality throughout the family. Samantha was able to say to her husband that his unavailability through travel and through his excessive drinking in the evenings left her alone and more focused on Adam, and that if he could improve those things, it would help her own attempt to be less suspiciously focused on Adam.

In this case, all three members of the family were able to own something about their own roles in provoking a breakdown of mutuality in the family. What they were discussing was the way that their link was contaminated from inside each of their minds and that this contaminated link then soured each of them psychically, so that they became more isolated, more depressed, more anxious internally, and more dissatisfied with one another – and more prone to live in their feared bad objects. Their capacity to improve by owning things themselves, by taking clear steps to improve their overt communication, and by sharing the mutuality of their disappointment and their wish to do better with each other led in a fairly easy way to dramatic improvement in the family.

The gains in the family were challenged six months later when Quentin discovered Adam smoking a joint one late night. In a return to family therapy, Adam insisted that this was only his second joint ever. He insisted that he had never smoked until that week. Quentin said that Adam looked pretty experienced and that he, Quentin, was not buying Adam's story. Samantha said that this, of course, set her back. What she wanted from the situation was that they not return to the "paranoid position" that she had previously brought to the family. I asked Quentin and Samantha about their own experience of smoking marijuana, which they then shared. Neither of their experiences was particularly remarkable in that neither of them had liked it, but they had both experimented in their adolescence. The three of them reviewed the improvement in their relationship that had previously ensued, and the parents were able to say that they were not so fixed now on stopping Adam from ever smoking marijuana, but much more on maintaining the restored trust that they had achieved. Adam agreed, and with implicit understanding that he would be likely to experiment further with marijuana, they were able to emerge from these sessions with regained trust.

Before giving a more extensive example, I want to add another central point about the way that the concept of the link helps with the concept of living in the object. So far, I have talked about the way our patients act as though they are living in an object inside themselves. They then externalize that psychic experience onto and into the people that they relate to.

But the concept of the link holds that there is an organization in the space between members of any emotional relationship that is unique to that couple, family or group. We can say that there are three organizations that make up any couple organization: (1) the psychic self-and-object organization of the first person; (2) the link between the two people or between members of the family; and (3) the introjection of the experience by the second person in resonance with the first person. In this third part, the first person is living inside the second subject as an indwelling internal object. These three organizations are each fractals of the totality of a complex dynamic pattern. In health the link between two people has dynamic resonance with the psychic self-and-object experience of each of the individuals. Inside each individual, a dynamic psychic structure oscillates among various self-and-object positions. It is only in the stasis of a fixed psychic structure that our patients come to act as though they are living almost literally within their inner objects. Then they project that sense of being inhabited onto the relationship the actual other person. In contrast, we consider it normal when parents live as though inside the mind of their children for periods of time. But in health, the parents can extricate themselves from that sense, can pull back to be external actual parents.

So, it is a matter of where the emotional emphasis is unconsciously assigned by the people involved, because each of us spends some time feeling as though we live in our internal objects. When we imagine ourselves inside the experience of our objects but then extricate ourselves to regain perspective so that we can experience the other person in the actual interaction, this is ordinary in-depth interaction with our important others. But when someone gets fixed and stuck, then we see a pathological situation. Therefore, it is a matter of where, in a person's fantasy, the person assigns the center of his or her psychic life and what flexibility the person has in moving from one position to another: In the self, in the link between the person and the other, or in the other person's mind.

My final example comes from an analysis carried out some years ago.

Audrey, a 40-year-old woman, had been in analysis for three years. She said that she had been cruelly treated by her parents, and most of her early material was about how she hated her mother. She also hated her father and wished that her parents would get on with dying even though they were nowhere near doing so. She organized her life unconsciously around taking revenge on them, which she had done by moving away, at their expense, and, over the first two years of treatment, not speaking to them. "Not speaking to them" is a relative matter in that she joined in the family chat, talked badly about them to her brother with whom she was on close terms, took money from them on occasion, and read her mother's occasional letters describing her mother's life and wishes for Audrey to be in active contact with her. She said that she did not talk much about her father because things were even worse with him. She said, "He sexualized his relationship with me when I was little. He didn't do anything frankly abusive, but there was a leer in his eye whenever he looked at me. I could feel him sizing me up sexually, getting off on anything sexual that he thought he saw. And he was emotionally abusive." Her most intensely ambivalent relationship, with alternating excitement and punishment, was with her grandfather, with whom she used to have sadomasochistic childhood games. She would taunt him and run away. He would give chase and spank her in a way that was simultaneously excitingly playful and sadistic. Nevertheless, he was the only figure she felt she had a positive relationship with.

On the day I am reporting from Audrey's analysis, we discussed her being stuck with anger and despair. All she could do was complain about her mother, and intersperse her hatred with saying to me, "You just don't get it!" This frequent complaint that I did not get it about how cruel her parents were to her led to her conviction that until and unless I did, nothing was going to change. She was not going to be able to give up her way of treating people cruelly herself that inevitably led to the feeling that nobody liked her. This was also true of her husband, who she felt was not a person she could ever feel passionately about, despite the fact that he treated her well, was endlessly loving, and stayed with her no matter how aggressively or dismissively she treated him.

In the session, I said to her that she had decided that her mother, too, had to "get it" before Audrey could ever change. She put control over her ability to effect change in another person: her mother, her husband, me. She said, "Do you think you can ever get it? That you can ever understand? Because you keep telling me that I shouldn't be so angry and mean." I said, "What I have said is, 'How long are you going to hold onto your anger?'" I said that in the past that she tried an endless number of maneuvers not to change: for instance, having a giddy approach to me at the beginning of the hours by turning onto her stomach to stare at me in a teasing way, knowing it annoyed me. She also tried being furious at me for not "getting it." But when these maneuvers did not work, she was slowly backed into having to face her anger. I said that she maintained her feeling that "no one gets it," and meanwhile she was nasty to all the important people in her life – her parents, colleagues and friends, husband, and me.

I said, "There is a stubborn clinging to your idea that the other person has to get it." She said, "I agree and I want my mother to get it because nothing can change until then." I said, "So the control of your happiness is in your mother's hands. It's a question of when will she ever get it, and you will never be able to change until she does."

"Never!" she said. "She'll never get it because she just doesn't understand how she was to me for all those years after she came back from abandoning me so she could go away to school."

I said, "So you have defined these things as impossible. Nothing will change because you put the control in her hands, or, now, in my hands." As I said this, I remembered that she had also taken her husband to me as a couple therapist in order to get me to change him. She had said in that first session that she thought I was the only person who could change him. He was not particularly interested in changing, and I soon realized that her effort to get me to change him was a substitute for any idea that she could change herself. When I had made this interpretation, it eventually led to her coming into analysis, but it had not ended her hopes of changing him.

She was now sobbing loudly. I said, "This is the sound of impossibility. No one will ever understand you. They will never change and therefore you can never change."

"It hurts so much. Why does it never go away no matter how much I cry? It's still there. I want to cut it out surgically. I cry every day. My grandfather killed himself because of it."

I said, "Tell me about that."

"He was angry, drinking and depressed. It got in his stomach. They cut his stomach out and I saw it. This big, round part was all green with mold on it. He was so angry. When they cleaned up our place, when we finally moved, I saw a picture of my grandfather and my grandmother in the '50s with my father and his brothers. I gave him the picture. He tore it up. I told my mother, and she said, 'I told you not to do that.' She meant I shouldn't have shown him the picture."

I said, "Now *you* wish that I wouldn't show you the pictures of what is happening inside yourself."

She said, "I don't care. What I care about is that you see these things. If I'm teasing you, it's that I'm only teasing you, and it's nothing else. You told me you didn't like that."

I said, "No. I said you were trying to avoid this kind of pain."

Audrey turned over on her back, in the position she had been in at the beginning of the hour. She pulled her coat to cover herself. I had always thought of this particular coat as being uncharacteristically masculine and stylistically harsh. She said, "I always cover myself with this coat because I can't stand being exposed. And my mother used to cover my belly button with a blanket because she thought cold air gets into you through your belly button. I just want to have some friends. There's no fun anywhere in my life."

Audrey lived in her bad objects. Her parents, grandparents, aunts, and uncles were nothing but bad objects to her. One of her brothers was a good object, the only one she was in close contact with, but his wife was another bad object because Audrey felt her to be in the way between Audrey and her idealized brother.

When a woman who lives so much in the world of her bad objects and inside the constraint of constant battle with these objects, we have to ask the question whether there are any good objects, and, if so, where are they? The answer is right there in front of me every day. Audrey had researched my life before seeking me out and continuing into treatment, more extensively than any patient I can remember. I was seeing her early in the days when everything about everybody first became discoverable through the Internet. She had looked up elements of my life and found pictures of me I did not know existed. Her fantasy life involved me in her sexual excitement with fantasies both of being included with me and being excluded by me in the painful replay of exclusion from her mother and from her parents' relationship. This intense daily focus on a fantasy ideal and idealized relationship with me supplanted any pleasure in the relationship with her husband. She had never had an actual boyfriend, even before marriage, with whom she could have a tangible romantic adolescent passion, the kind that could organize an idealized relationship that would contribute to the destruction of the ideal parental relationship and therefore to ordinary resolution of Oedipal idealization. Instead, she had a lifelong search for an unobtainable idealized figure who would save her. By offering her analysis, I had offered to take on the role of that savior – and therefore to become inevitably guilty of failing to save her and thereby of failing her idealization. In these times I became the object of her rage, the same disappointment afforded by her mother and, in the more painfully unspeakable ways, her father. All of this boiled down to her formula that "You just don't get it." So, when the idealization failed, her ability to live in the idealized fantasy object crashed to the earth. She was not only let down; she was furious.

On the following day, Audrey described how, since the beginning of their relationship, she had not been able to feel excited sexually with her husband, because when he would touch her, she would connect the experience to being molested and would feel molestation was occurring now. But last evening, she had felt some small sexual excitement for the first time with him. She had an accompanying fantasy: "I was being tied down and couldn't move. I was being stimulated by an ugly, disgusting old man, against my will and I found it exciting. Then I had a fantasy about wanting revenge, which I also found exciting."

A few days later she discussed more about something she had never told me that she found exciting. "I thought about a fantasy of you and my couple therapist sexually. My family is so violent. My husband needs for me to offer him softness and gentleness, which I can't give him. My fantasy about our couple therapist is that she's just so soft and gentle. That gives me a lot of sexual excitement, just her talking, not actually being sexual herself. There are so many things that she likes that I like. [She had extensively researched the couple therapist as well.] She's curious and intelligent. My mother was contemptuous about me wanting to read interesting things like philosophy. She said to me 'Why would you want to read that? Are you going to make money from it? It's useless.' But I can see that my couple therapist is a widely read woman."

I said, "You feel critical of me for not wanting to hear how bored you are with your husband."

She said, "That's true. You want me to discuss my role in the boring relationship." She went on to describe how her mother was boring, too. Well maybe not *that* boring, because her mother had encouraged her to dance, which she likes very much. But then her mother would want to discuss only how she should compete. At this point she went back to talking about her husband being boring. I pointed out that she'd settled back into talking about him being boring instead of the idea of having to develop herself in order to keep herself from being boring. During this discussion she finally was able to talk about how she had offloaded the need to change herself onto him instead of considering the possibility she could change herself. I said that this was because she was convinced it was a hopeless project to think of changing herself.

She said, "That's right. I blame him for not having a social life when I don't. I blame him for things I can't do myself either. I know I have to do that for myself instead of compelling him to change. I have to leave him alone."

I said, "That's a change, from blaming him and hoping to change him because you can't change, to saying you know that's what you have to do yourself."

"Yes, but I still don't think you get how boring he is. Really, really boring! Which he has been from the beginning. But it's okay. I have to stop looking outside and start working on myself."

I said, "Do you think you picked him because, since he wasn't exciting sexually, he made you feel safe? Because in that case, he would never threaten to sexualize you like your father or grandfather or look at you with your father's leer? That way he would be safe, at the price of being sexually exciting."

She turned on her stomach, giggling, and said, looking at me, "It's so funny how boring he is." But then she said she had pulled back from wanting to divorce him, to now realizing how good he had been to her. That realization was forcing her to look into herself. It was a realization that put pressure on her to grow.

I said, "Do you think you feel anyone can ever love you?"

"No," she said. "I don't feel I'm lovable. But he loves me anyway. But then I can't love him, partly because I feel he doesn't see how bad I am, so he actually doesn't get me."

A few minutes later, she said, "I hate you! No! I don't really hate you, but you're too strict. You make me do things I don't want to do."

In this segment Audrey moved from a position of hopelessness about whether she could ever change, as expressed over many months of *living in* her intractably boring, hopelessly unchanging husband-object, to now beginning to consider the possibility of changing herself. This led me to ask, and her to say, that she felt fundamentally unlovable. In this process, we can see that she had been inhabiting people who expressed her ideal fantasy, but in more realistic ways than her habitual fantasy way of living in her idealized object in order to offset how she lived so much in hated internal objects. And, in the transference, she began to develop a fantasy couple that is connected to her fantasy idealized woman. There was now an oscillation between her sadomasochistic fantasy that had been part of the hated objects she lived in, the fantasy objects she was now creating, and a slight hint of a move toward a more realistic ideal object that might guide her to a different way of living. Finally, we hear that at the bottom of her need to live in her objects was the feeling that she was fundamentally unlovable and was hopeless about ever being able to love or be loved. This realization presaged later stages for us in her analysis.

Conclusion

Living in the object is a common part of everyday life in which we imagine ourselves inside the mind of people who are important to us. We do so inside our own minds. But in health, we are able to pull back, to extricate ourselves, to form a link of mutual give-and-take, to repair periods of misunderstanding. The repair of understanding between people who can see themselves as separate persons and who communicate aspects of their inner world to each other through their interpersonal links can then inform the development of each of them (Scharff and Scharff, 2011). In the form of illness that I have been describing, persons get stuck in their own minds inside their inner objects, whether it be an object of idealization and excessive love, or an object of hatred and mutual attack. In these cases, it is as though nothing we do could help unless we agree to help them change their objects. These patients think it is not helpful to change their own perspective, their own minds. We are pressed to change their actual object.

I should have picked up on this more than 30 years ago when one of my patients said to me, "I have finally realized that I'm here to have you cure my parents." This is a common position for many patients, but fortunately most of them are eventually willing to move on to examination of the organization of their own minds. Only after the realization that their own growth cannot be contingent on changing the people in their lives can they be free them to do difficult work on themselves.

References

Fairbairn, W. R. D. (1952). *Psychoanalytic Studies of the Personality*. London: Routledge and Kegan Paul.

Losso, R., de Setton, L. and Scharff, D. E. (Eds.) (2017). *The Linked Self in Psychoanalysis: The Pioneering Work of Enrique Pichon Rivière*. London & New York: Karnac.

Scharff, D. E., Losso, R. and Setton, L. (2017). Pichon-Rivière's psychoanalytic contributions: Some comparisons with object relations and modern developments in psychoanalysis. *International Journal of Psychoanalysis*, 98(1): 129–143.

Scharff, D. E. and Scharff, J. S. (2011). *The Interpersonal Unconscious*. Lanham, MD: Jason Aronson.

Winnicott, D. W. (1971). The use of an object and relating through identifications. In *Playing and Reality*. London: Tavistock, pp. 86–94.

2 What does the object (in our patients' lives) have to do with it?

James L. Poulton

To set the stage

I begin by quoting the Bodhidharma from the sixth century CE:

> Then for the first time I dwelled upright in dark quiescence and settled external objects in the kingdom of mind. . . . For the first time I realized that within the square inch of my own mind there is nothing that does not exist.
>
> (Broughton, 1999, p. 12)

I would like to approach psychoanalytic objects by considering the role of external objects in our patient's lives and even in our patient's minds. Let me start with a seemingly unrelated observation.

One of the central events that led to the capture of Ted Kaczynski (a serial killer, nicknamed the Unabomber, who was at large for 17 years) was a psycholinguistic analysis of the 35,000-word manifesto he mailed to the *New York Times*. The analysis concluded that because the manifesto contained terms used by newspapers from Chicago in the 1930s, '40s, and '50s, the Unabomber was most likely raised in that area. Because of the analysis, the FBI decided to publish the manifesto, with the hope that someone would be able to link its language to its author. Shortly thereafter, Kaczynski's brother and sister-in-law contacted the FBI and provided additional letters and documents they had received from him, which ultimately led to his capture (Davies, 2017).

The interesting part of this story, for our purposes, is that the Unabomber's actions could not help but reveal the traces of the social/interpersonal environments in which he had developed and which had inscribed in him specific characteristics that he thereafter exhibited as evidence of their influence. In an important sense, this story reveals that external objects are in some way *inherent* in us.

The question, however, is this: In *what way* is the object inherent in us? What does it mean to say that we bear the traces of the object within us? And then, depending on what we decide about the role of the object in our lives, what implications does it have for how we treat our patients?

Psychoanalysis and the external object

For many years, psychoanalysis has had a lot to say about *internal* objects and the role they play in shaping everything about us. Recently, however, psychoanalytic theorists have begun to focus more on *external* objects and to explore whether they influence our experience and behavior in ways that are different from the influence of the internal objects with which we are more familiar.

The question I would like to consider, then, pertains to the role the real, external object may play in our patients' lives, apart from how they have internalized those objects. I have in mind a particular situation in which a patient attends sessions with us but then returns to a relationship with another person who has been instrumental in generating some or most of our patient's pathological adaptations. A characteristic example is the case of a young man, Damien, whom I will introduce in more detail later, who developed a pattern of extremely harsh treatment of himself as a way to calm his harsh and judgmental mother. Following some of my meetings with this patient, he would call his mother to discuss our session. When I would meet him for the next session, I would feel that we had lost the ground we had gained and that we had to cover again the same territory we had already traversed. Although this phase did not last through all of the treatment, while it was occurring I felt as if I was in a tug of war over the patient: I and my views were on one side, and his mother and her pathological influence over her son were on the other.

Before I get to the case, though, I propose a quick tour of some of the theories that have led to a re-examination of the external object and its place in the life of the individual. I merely wish to get a few basic ideas under our belts, enough to help us frame the discussion of how to deal with Damien and his mother.

The intersubjective vs. the intrapsychic

With the rise of such theories as intersubjectivity, relationality, the analytic third, the analytic field, and the vínculo or Link, analysts have explored two primary dimensions of psychic experience: the intrapsychic and the interactive or "interpsychic" (Bolognini, 2004). The chief concerns of most of these writers have been, first, to illuminate the differences between these two dimensions, and, second, to describe the ways in which the two interact and jointly or mutually influence each other.

Pichon-Rivière, for example, suggested these two dimensions jointly interact to create what he called the Link. Through the idea of the Link, Pichon-Rivière "attempted to explore the complex relationship between the way that external object relations influence internal organization throughout life, and in turn, how internal object relations organize external interaction" (Scharff, 2009, p. 69; see also Losso, de Setton and Scharff, 2017).

Berenstein (2001, 2009, 2012) and Kaës (1995, 2007) were also concerned with developing the concept of the Link. Berenstein (2009), for example, followed Pichon-Rivière in suggesting that a Link is produced by two different mechanisms: "a predominantly individual mechanism" based on each participant's internal object relationships that function in interactions "by means of projective identification" and an "in-between" mechanism in which the real-time interaction between the participants exerts its own pressure – outside the participants' internal object relations – on the course of the interaction. This second "in-between" mechanism is the result of what Berenstein calls "interference" (2009, p. 86).

Berenstein believed that who we are is the result of two kinds of investments by others in our development. The first is through the process of *identification*, in which the other serves as a model for what we *want* to be. Through this process we establish internalized, symbolizable aspects of the object that thereafter guide our experience and behavior. The second process, in contrast, occurs through acts of *interference*, according to which we *have* to adapt to the other because we have encountered something in them "which resists and cannot be incorporated" (2001, p. 145). This process is distinct from object relations (2009, p. 86) and is something that we cannot represent to ourselves (2012, p. 574). A possible example of interference: you have just finished an evaluative interview with a prospective patient who has, unbeknownst to you, a repressed history of trauma in relationship with her father, and you realize afterward that you forgot to ask about the father. In this case, an unrepresented part of the patient may have interfered with your capacity to think, without your knowing how or why the interference occurred.

Berenstein refers to the aspect of the other that "resists and cannot be incorporated" as *alien* or *foreign* (2012) and emphasizes that its impact on us is a consequence of being in the here-and-now *presence* of the other. When we interact with another, there will be part of the person with which we *can* identify and that fits easily into our internal object world. But there will be another, alien part that will *not* fit easily into our internal world because we will have no way of representing it. It is this part of the other that *interferes* with the ordinary flow of our experience.

When Berenstein turns his attention to the interactions between therapist and patient, he again speaks of two dimensions or "modalities" (2009). The first is the modality of *transference*, in which the patient's internal object world is repeated or reproduced in relationship to the therapist. The key aspect of this modality is that the experiences that generated the patient's internal world can be worked through via careful attention to the here-and-now of the session and the there-and-then of the patient's past. For the second modality Berenstein again uses the term "interference," but in this case interference – especially that imposed on the patient by the therapist – can be used for positive gain, since through it therapist and patient can generate new and potentially healthier experiences by making "a space for the otherness of the other subject" (2009, p. 88). In Janine Puget's terms, interference can make room "for surprise, for a form of belonging that does not fit into the set of problems tied to identity" (2012, p. 786). Because of its growth-enhancing potential, Berenstein regarded interference as equal to transference, in terms of its efficacy in bringing about change, and repeatedly stated that "we need to work therapeutically with both of them" (2009, p. 87).

The French psychoanalyst Rene Kaës is another writer who has made substantial contributions to the theory of the Link (1993, 1995, 1998, 2007; Kirshner, 2006). Like Pichon-Rivière and Berenstein, Kaës recognizes that the other influences us either through the internalization of representable aspects of the other (which become bound "to our own private ends" Kirshner, 2006, p. 1006) or through the transmission of something foreign, "an obscure and unknown presence of another . . . inside [the self]," which functions as "a kind of unassimilated other dwelling as a permanent guest, unwelcome or unknown, within the psyche" (Kaës, 1993, p. 5, translated by and quoted in Kirshner, 2006, p. 1006).

For Kaës, this "indwelling" of the other as an unassimilated, unknown guest in our psyche is a significant source of psychopathology. Kaës speaks of the "requirement of psychic work imposed by the subjectivity of the object" (1995, p. 2) on the self and says that the content or meaning of these requirements may never be represented – either by ourselves or by the object. When they are imposed on us, however, they lead to what Kaës terms "diseases of intersubjective contracts" (p. 2), which include "agreements" to participate in mutual acts of repression, erasure, denial, splitting, and misunderstanding or refusals to know and which result in areas of non-signifiability and non-transformability, "zones of silence," "pockets of intoxication," "garbage spaces," and "lines of flight that keep the subject a stranger to her own history" (1995, p. 13). From Kaës's perspective, these requirements "inscribe" themselves on us, and our experience and behavior are thereafter modified or conditioned by the presence of those inscriptions, whether or not we remain in the presence of the original object.

Some of you might have noticed a point of disagreement between Berenstein and Kaës in what I have written. Berenstein says that the alien parts of the other influence a person only when the two are actually interacting in the here and now, but Kaës says that "diseases of intersubjective contracts" can modify a person's psychic activity even after the original interactions have ceased. In this respect, Kaës's position is similar to that of Gabbard, who says he believes, contrary to Berenstein, that Links and their pathological effects "persist in spite of physical separation" (2012, p. 585). This is an issue we will return to when we consider the case of Damien.

Kaës's language may be new to us, but I would suggest that diseases of intersubjective contracts are quite common in our patients and have been identified by other theorists under a variety of names, including "schemas of being-with" (Stern, 1995), "implicit relational knowing" (Lyons-Ruth, 1999; Stern et al., 1998), "relational scripts" (Trevarthen, 1993), and "the haunting of the phantom" (Abraham and Torok, 1994). A good example of these diseases can be found in Abraham and Torok's description of a family in which a traumatized mother has so deeply repressed her trauma that she is unaware of its nature or its distorting effects on her emotional and behavioral functioning. In such a family, the growing child adapts to her mother's distortions, participates in them, and even supports her mother in the exercise of such distortions, but *without understanding their purpose or origin*. This process, in turn, saddles the child with fears that have no images to ground them, behavioral patterns with no apparent meaning, and "blank spots" in her mind where thoughts cannot be thought, emotions cannot be felt, and desires cannot be acknowledged. Abraham and Torok call this process the haunting of the phantom, the hallmark of which is that the child becomes invaded by an alien presence whose meaning lies not in the child's own experience but in the details of the mother's trauma (cf. Poulton, 2013).

Therapeutic strategies for diseases of intersubjective contracts

The theories I have just reviewed raise some vexing questions about psychoanalytic technique. Suppose a patient enters therapy and you discover that aspects of his experience and behavior are, as Kaës and Berenstein describe, unassimilated into his internal object world and are therefore neither signifiable nor representable. Suppose further that you suspect these characteristics in the patient are the result of diseases of intersubjective contracts that have taken hold in the patient because he is still in thrall to a close relationship, such as with a mother or spouse. What kinds of interventions will help to dislodge these contracts and free the patient from the limitations imposed on him? What interventions are useful when working with unrepresented influences over the patient?

One thing theorists of the Link agree upon is that traditional transference analysis, while still centrally important, is not sufficient when the patient's problems arise from Links with others. Berenstein, for example, believed that because transference analysis is primarily focused on *representable* aspects of the patient's internal world, it overlooks mechanisms of interference and their consequences. Similarly, Kaës has written that intersubjective contracts "cannot be reduced to a taking into consideration of the place and function of the Other and the others in intrapsychic space" (1998, p. 4; quoted by Kirshner, 2006, p. 1012). José Bleger, another theorist of the Link, wrote that an exclusive focus on here-and-now transference "may lead to blind spots about external vínculos [Links] that are problematic in other domains of the patient's daily life" (Gabbard, 2012, p. 583).

Gabbard elaborates on Bleger's point, saying that most patients "at some point recognize that they have lived their lives to please" or to "avoid the wrath, criticism, or humiliation of someone else" and that "*the very essence of analytic working through is to identify these linkages as they emerge in the transference and outside the transference in order to shed light on who we actually are in light of these linkages and in spite of them*" (2012, p. 584, emphasis added).

Helping a patient understand who he is "in light of these linkages and in spite of them" requires, of course, that the therapist investigate how and why the relationships in his life function the way they do. And this, in turn, requires that the treatment sometimes focus not so much on the patient but on the motives, needs, and pathologies of the external objects surrounding him that have played a role in binding the patient in his diseases of intersubjective contracts. Indeed, it is only through such a focus on external objects that the therapist can follow Gabbard's recommendation or those of Thomä and Kächele, who said the therapist "must, in collaboration with the patient, provide him insights into his situation in life"

(1992, p. 482) or those of Lemma and Target, who said the therapist "takes the many opportunities provided by the patient's description of real-life interpersonal incidents to help the patient to exercise flexible understanding of the possible feelings and thoughts (of the different individuals involved), getting the patient to elaborate different internal scenarios perhaps underlying these incidents, questioning habitual assumptions" (2011, p. 156). The danger, of course, is that focusing on the patient's external objects can potentially imbalance the treatment to the point of losing sight of the patient's own contributions to creating and maintaining problematic patterns. Consideration of the case of Damien will help us explore the reasonable limits to the effectiveness of such interventions.

Before we get to Damien, though, two other intervention strategies that address diseases of intersubjective contracts deserve mention. First, it is of utmost importance that we recognize that transference analysis should not automatically be ejected when working with such "diseases." Stern and colleagues have made this important point in an article on non-interpretive mechanisms in analytic therapy. They suggest that a patient's "implicit relational" patterns that are "not symbolically represented but are not necessarily dynamically unconscious" (1998, p. 905) can be brought to light in treatment through transference interpretations of the way the patient *behaves* with the therapist. Stern et al. are making a subtle but important point. Not all transference arises from identifiable or symbolizable internal objects in the patient's internal world. Instead, some transferences will consist in a non-represented, non-symbolized repetition of behaviors and patterns of experience the patient has come to embody in the intersubjective contracts the patient has with others. This, I believe, is especially the case when those behaviors and patterns of experience are held in place by a current relationship in the patient's daily life.

The final intervention strategy refers us back to Berenstein's and Puget's idea that the therapist can function as a source of interference for the patient in a way that helps the patient not only in "making room for the other as a different subject" (Berenstein, 2012, p. 576) but also in allowing him- or herself to participate in the therapeutic relationship "in so far as it has the potential to create and shape both a subject and new ideas" (Puget, 2006, p. 1697). This point is emphasized by Scharff, who says that the therapist, by his or her presence, can work as a "destabilizing force" (2009, p. 82) in the patient's basic patterns of interaction. This is to say that the therapist's presence, as a (one hopes) non-pathological participant in a growing Link with the patient, exerts a form of unsymbolized and perhaps unsymbolizable pressure on the patient that helps the patient disengage from the constraints imposed by relationships with external objects. Certainly, much more can be said about this particular form of intervention with our patients, but it is time now to turn to Damien.

Damien

I met Damien three and a half years ago. He was 29 years old and in his third year of a very demanding graduate program. Because of his schedule, we could not meet on a consistent basis: sometimes we were unable to meet for two or three weeks in a row, followed by one or two weeks when we would meet up to three times per week. This pattern persisted throughout our two and a half years together. Our work ended when he finished his degree, got married, and took a job in another state.

Damien was the second oldest of four children, all born within one or two years of each other. Although he didn't talk often of his three sisters, the one he spoke most about was his next younger sister, who had been bulimic and anorexic from the age of 18 and had spent "many months" in various institutions for what he called "borderline" behaviors. Damien described his parents as very religious and devoted to their religious community. Despite their devotion, they would not infrequently get into violent fights in which they "lost control" and which "absolutely terrified" him. His mother, he said, was rigid, judgmental, and unforgiving: "She says what she thinks as she thinks it. She has a strong personality." Damien attributed his mother's rigid religiosity to a "history of mental health issues," including bulimia in her teens, extreme anxiety throughout her life, and enduring guilt about an abortion she had in her twenties before marrying his father. Damien blamed most of the difficulties of his childhood on his mother and saw his father as calmer and more forgiving. His father, he said, was "passive" "thoughtful," "hard on himself," someone who "takes care of other people first." When Damien was young, he and his father went on fishing trips together, but as Damien got older their relationship became more distant as his father spent more time at work.

Damien was home-schooled until high school because his parents objected to public schools for religious reasons. Between the ages of about four and ten, he said, he "at least" had a group of friends who understood and accepted him. When he was ten, however, his parents moved the family to a new city, and from then on he felt isolated and ostracized by other children because of his family's beliefs. This was the reason, he believed, that he "wasn't a socially comfortable kid." From the age of ten, he said, he hated his parents, both because of the move and because he "got the shit kicked out of me a lot" by his mother while his father did little to intervene. His mother, he said, was extremely critical of him, would often beat him with a belt, and rarely attempted to understand his perspective. He believed his mother hated males and that she took her wrath out on him because his father was often absent.

For a "significant portion" of his adolescence, Damien had a suicide plan, and he came close to attempting suicide on multiple occasions. He said the main theme of his suicidal thoughts was "the conviction that nobody loves me and nobody can love me." When he left home to go to college, he immediately stopped attending church, and in our second session he said, "I have this visceral reaction to religion now that's a function of my growing up."

Before his move to Salt Lake City, where I met him, Damien was in treatment with a psychoanalyst who helped him explore "traumas that gave me a poor self-concept. He said as my brain matured it looked for ways to justify my negative self-perception." As he and I began treatment, Damien described multiple symptoms of depression and anxiety, including severe and persistent self-negation and devaluation, social isolation, and avoidance of any situation in which he might be judged. For example, he refused to open letters of evaluation from his graduate supervisors for six months, and he delayed writing an assigned report for more than a year. Given that his program was quite prestigious, and given that his overall presentation was one of a capable and intelligent young man, the unrealistic nature of the attacks he launched against himself was all the more disturbing. As treatment progressed, we linked his self-devaluation – his certainty about his badness – both to his enduring anger at his mother (being not-good-enough, we agreed, was a way of being angry with his mother without being aware of his anger) and to the pressure he felt from her to accept her attacks without complaint, even agree with them, as the price he had to pay to minimize their intensity.

I would like to briefly describe four sessions I had with Damien. The first three are contiguous and occurred near the end of the second year of treatment. In these sessions, we discussed the nature of the unacknowledged agreements, à la Kaës, he had reached with his mother that led to his pattern of harsh self-judgment. It was during this time that Damien was in fairly steady contact with his mother. The fourth session, which occurred several months later, near the end of treatment, focused on his transferential attempts to enlist me in his self-attacks and his difficulty doing so because he found me to be an "uncooperative" partner. When viewed from the perspective of Berenstein, Puget, and Scharff, Damien's difficulty with me stemmed from my having presented an intersubjective pressure (i.e., interference) on him that pressured him to disengage from the self-limiting patterns imposed by his relationship with his mother.

Three sessions at end of second year

Damien began the first of these sessions saying he was frustrated with his progress and thought he should be working faster. He added that he was not working faster because he was a "lazy-ass procrastinator" who never did anything he should. I commented that the spontaneity and forcefulness of his attack on himself suggested there was something he was afraid of. He agreed and said that throughout his life he had been afraid he wouldn't be loved or valued or esteemed. "I feel my fear was fairly evidence based," he said. "My mother was mad at me so often. And when I did incur her wrath, I felt I had done *bad* on a fundamental level. When her punishment was physical, I didn't feel it as discipline – it felt like an attack. . . . When I erred, it was in terms of biblical and godly standards – I had sinned and fallen short of the glory of god." "Your badness was biblical," I said, "because your mother needed goodness to be biblical as well?" Damien then talked of a phone call with his mother a few days earlier. She had talked about *her* father – how he had been extremely demanding and unstinting in his criticisms if she failed to live up to his standards. "My mother had the idea," he said, "that we had to match up to a standard, to rise above her upbringing. She had a need for achievement, for looking good for her father. For her father, value was earned, not given." "And she brought the same pattern to you?" I asked. "For me," Damien said, "my mother's unhappiness was linked to some form of doom – something that would lead to her anger, which for me was a disaster. So, we kids started to monitor her unhappiness. We got good at it." "You monitored it in order to try to repair it?" I asked. Damien said, "In my childhood, nothing was ever done *enough* – the house was never clean enough, the garden was never weeded enough, I never did anything fast enough. It wasn't so much terrifying as it was depressing. I remember feeling, all the time, *this will never get any better*." At this, Damien began to cry, which embarrassed him and led him to say something about how stupid he was to be crying. I said, "I think what has just happened is important. You've covered up your pain – about the fear and hopelessness you felt as a child – with yet another self-attack. I imagine that's what you did as a child, and I imagine it worked, not just for you, but for your mother too." Damien said, "You mean it's okay to cry? I'm not being stupid?" I was struck by how young this question made Damien sound, but I only shook my head to say, no, it wasn't stupid. He said, "When I was three or four, I would be devastated if I colored outside the lines. Being ashamed of myself feels like the natural order of things. If at three I was anxious because my mother was, then conformity was the solution to both our anxieties." "All of these brutal and harsh things you say about yourself," I said, "function as a way of *not* thinking about something else – how injured, sad, and hopeless you felt. And it sounds like that *not-thinking* worked both for you and your mother. I wonder if that's what you mean by the 'natural order of things.'"

Damien began our next session, five days later, by telling me he hadn't been doing well. "I had some evenings off," he said, "and I didn't do anything. I didn't study, I didn't write, I didn't even go out with friends. I just sat around beating myself up for being such a lazy bastard." He then talked about how he had disappointed a program supervisor because he was "too stupid to answer a basic question," and how he was too fat because he is "so lazy I won't even do what I know is good for me." I said, "The part of you that needs to berate you is out in full force today. I wonder why." After some back and forth about whether his self-contempt was overstating its case, Damien grew silent. After a long moment, he said, "I called my mother last night. I was telling her I was lonely. She said 'You need an attitude of gratitude.' It's from a f***ing kid's song! She throws a f***ing kid's song at me! I've been lonely since I was ten." I said, "I suspect there's a connection between your phone call and the intensity in your self-contempt as you began today." Damien said, "You mean she devalued me by quoting the kid's song, and I then devalued myself?" I said, "Yes, there's that. But it feels to me like there's something else. Something like: you were hurt by your mother's inability to respond to your real feelings of loneliness, but then forgot about being hurt by putting extra energy into attacking yourself." Damien said, "Now I'm feeling guilty about being angry at her. She's done the best she could. She's even apologized to me for how she treated me as a kid. Why can't I get over it and accept her apology?" I said, "There it is again. You're using self-devaluation to beat back anger and pain. The self-devaluation essentially says 'Get over it already – I don't want to hear about it.'" Damien: "I guess my mom's response to pain was to say 'get over it' in a lot of different ways – 'attitude of gratitude,' 'God will take care of it' – I guess that was somewhat difficult, given that she was also the source of the pain."

Because of Damien's schedule, the next session occurred two weeks later. Damien began by saying that after our prior session, he had been depressed and found himself obsessing about his "failures." "But then I pulled myself together and did a reasonable job of telling myself I'm not as bad as I think I am." He then said, "I talked to my mom. I told her I'm trying to reconcile her with the 'old' mom. She understood. I said I was still angry at the old mom. I was whining a bit. She said something about, 'That's where grace comes in,' and I just blew up. I don't need that 'attitude of gratitude' shit." I said, "It's difficult for your mom to be present to your pain." Damien said, "I was saying I don't know if this will ever get better or if this will ever get fixed, *and God comes along*!" I said, "You mean your mother turned to God instead of you when she made the comment about grace?" Damien: "I think I wanted something from her and what she offered instead was something that has hurt me in the past. Between the ages of 10 and about 14, I was probably hoping God would intervene in my hating myself. But by 15 I was in a 'f*** God' mood. F*** that shit, it wasn't f***ing real. I truly detest the church. It's about looking good, a keeping-up-with-appearances attitude." I said, "Your anger at the church is rooted in how injured you are by a move your mother continues to make. It's a move that lifts your conversation with her out of the human level and into an abstract level – where the interaction is about God and no longer about your injury, or how you feel or how you are doing. It's a move that places her out of your reach." Damien then told me that his mother had been raised Catholic but later got involved in the evangelical Christian tradition. He said he thought evangelism offered his mother a chance at her own redemption from the "terrible guilt" she felt over her past. He then said, "The 14-year-old me was an ashamed, depressed, suicidal, angry, lonely person. So, my parents turned me over to God and all I got there was judgment for nonconformity." I said, "The 14-year-old you was in a lot of pain." As Damien took some time to respond, I watched his face harden. Where there had been sadness, there was now contempt. He said, "The 14-year-old me: what I think is that he's a little bitch. I'm embarrassed at a lot of his behavior." I said, "And there's another repetition of the sequence from anger and pain to self-attack." Damien said, "If I stop blaming the 14-year-old, all that's left is feeling sad about all this. I'd be overwhelmed by a sea of sadness." At this he began crying again, although he tried to hide it by wiping tears away as quickly as they appeared. After a pause, I said, "This is the sadness you hide from yourself by covering it with self-blame." Damien: "If I go into that sea of sadness I don't know if I'll come up. If I go into it, I'll feel contempt for myself. Maybe I can tell myself, 'the grief you have is reasonable, understandable, real. There's nothing aberrant about having it.'" I nodded. The session was over.

When working with a patient whose behavior has been influenced by an unsymbolized and unacknowledged "contract" with another person, particularly one who is still active in the patient's life, the therapist's role must shift in some significant ways. In the sessions described earlier, my intent was to weave together the patterns I witnessed in Damien during our sessions with the real-life dynamics of his relationship with his mother. To that end, my focus alternated between the here-and-now of the session, the there-and-then of his past relationship with his mother, and the "there-and-now" of his current interactions with her that had immediate effects on his behavior and attitudes toward himself. By doing so, I was trying to symbolize what had never been symbolized by or for Damien: the real parameters of his unconscious agreement with his mother that both parties remain unaware of the pain, sadness, and anger he felt through much of his life. Those parameters included his mother's fear and guilt, her need to deny her contributions to her children's distress, and Damien's complementary need to rescue her from her anxieties. If Damien was going to emerge from the "disease" this unconscious agreement had induced in him, it would be through his explicit understanding of these parameters and through his subsequent working through of the painful realities of both his past and his present.

In the following session, which occurred near the end of treatment, our focus had shifted. Instead of illuminating the foundations of his agreement with his mother (as in the three sessions already described), we turned to exploring how that agreement had influenced Damien's relationship with me. Our conversations at this point occurred in the two different modalities I have already described. First, we explicitly discussed Damien's assumptions about himself and about me that led him to attempt to perpetuate, in the transference, the basic structures of his agreement with his mother. These interactions fell within the boundaries of traditional analysis of transference, since they focused on what was, by this point, representable and symbolizable in Damien's psyche. The second modality conformed to Berenstein's concept of therapeutic interference, in the sense that I resisted the (countertransferential) pressure on me to play the same role as Damien's mother and instead presented him with an alternative way of being with another person – one in which he did not have to replace his self-awareness with self-attack. By the end of this session, as a result of my refusal to conform to past patterns, Damien was experiencing some confusion as to what role he *might* play with me. This state, which has been described by Beier and Young as an experience of "beneficial uncertainty" (1998, p. 65), is a precursor to therapeutic change because it implies that the pressures underlying old patterns have weakened to the point that new arrangements are now possible.

Fourth session

Over the next several months, Damien and I continued our irregular meeting schedule. During this time, I saw significant progress: he attacked himself less frequently, and when he did he was increasingly able to question his motives for doing so. He began dating a woman he met at school, and he began talking about his growing affection for her. The following session occurred after I had been on a two-week break when he otherwise would have been able to meet with me.

Damien began by saying, "While you were gone, I did get a few things done, but none without dragging myself to it. Basically, I was lazy." "You were lazy," I said, in a tone that said I was aware he was devaluing himself again. He said, "I can't tell you how many hours I wasted saying to myself, 'What are you doing, you lazy piece of shit?'" I said, "It sounds like you're comforting yourself by reminding yourself of your badness. As you've said many times, it's how you guarantee your place in the order of things." Damien thought for a moment and said, "Almost what I'm doing is affirming my avoidance – recognizing that it's a valid strategy that I've used in the past." I said, "I guess the question is, avoidance of what?" He said, "I don't really know." I paused, then said, "I suspect you do." He said, "What do you mean?" I said, "Well, for one thing, I've been away for two weeks when we might have met, and we're coming up on the time that you'll be done with your training and leaving Salt Lake. Maybe you have some feelings about it." Damien was silent for at least a couple of minutes. He then said, "I'm not sure I have a right to miss you." "You missed me," I said. Damien nodded almost imperceptibly and became interested in his hands. He was wearing a sweatshirt and he pulled the hoodie over his head. I said, "I see that it feels like something needs to be hidden – something like sadness?" Damien said, after another pause, "I am sad. I'm sad that we're going to stop meeting." I said, "I wonder if you're also angry with me because I arranged my break so we couldn't meet these past two weeks." Damien: "If I don't have a right to miss you. I definitely don't have a right to be angry with you." I said, "I think the old sequence has kicked in between you and me. I hurt you. . . ." At this, Damien shook his head but didn't say anything. I said, "Okay, I know it's hard to acknowledge it, but . . . I hurt you, and you're sad and angry about it. But the old sequence between you and your mother told you it was part of the order of things to hide those feelings, from me and from yourself. So, you accomplished that by telling me you've been a lazy piece of shit." Damien said, "It's how I've always defined myself." I said, "Defined and protected yourself. And I think you're trying to protect me, too." Damien said, "I suppose it could be that I'm not certain how to define myself beyond that." I said, "I think you're saying that it hasn't been in your basic repertoire how to talk with someone who has hurt you, and still expect them to want to listen." Damien said, "I talked with my mother last week. She told me that when she was 21, she had an epiphany that 'God does not make junk.' I took it to mean that she felt suddenly valuable – *absolutely* valuable – and that was a solution to the conditional value she felt in the eyes of her father. But then I thought: If she was suddenly valuable in the eyes of God, then where did all her guilt go? I think she needed us kids to be perfect so she could prove to God that *she* was. And when we weren't, she blamed us." I said, "Accepting that blame was a way of saving your mother from her fears. And because those fears were so strong, you couldn't talk about how the whole arrangement was hurting you. This morning, by beginning with an attack on yourself, you were doing the same thing with me." Damien said, "Yeah, but it's harder to do it with you – you don't give me any of that God shit." I said, "And you don't quite know what to do with that." Damien said, "Right, I don't know what to do with it."

Conclusion

I would like to make a few observations about the nature of intersubjective contracts and the methods by which they can be treated:

1 As I mentioned earlier, there is a fairly clear divergence between the way Kaës and Berenstein understand the kinds of pathological influence the "alien" parts of one person can have on another. Their divergence centers around whether such influence can persist even when the two are separated. The case of Damien seems to help settle this debate: Although Damien's mother was never physically present in our sessions, her influence over his experience and behavior was substantial and undeniable.
2 The influence Damian's mother had over him was sustained and reinforced by the frequent telephone contact between the two. From one perspective, their conversations can be viewed as analogous to mutual hypnotic inductions, in which each reminded the other, without knowing they were doing so, of the nature and parameters of their basic agreement.
3 It is important to recognize that the unconscious agreement Damien reached with his mother was most likely instigated, initially, by *her* relationship trauma with her father, whose "unstinting criticisms" seem to have been instrumental in the development of rigid, black-and-white defenses that found their full expression in the fervor of her religious beliefs. This observation, in turn, raises two additional points. First, a pathological relationship between two people will always be embedded within and supported by a matrix of *other* relationships – with past generations, with current familial and social groups, and even with broader societal and cultural institutions. This point was forcefully made by Pichon-Rivière (Losso, de Setton and Scharff, 2017). Second, it is possible to regard some diseases of intersubjective contracts as special cases of the intergenerational transmission of trauma. This is especially the case when a parent's defenses against trauma are both rigidly oriented toward denial and when the child is enlisted early in life to participate in the parent's will to not know about his or her own trauma in order to rescue the parent from overwhelming anxiety.
4 The case of Damien illustrates that treatment of a patient constrained by an intersubjective contract may require the therapist to go beyond the therapeutic modes of interference and transference analysis in order to interpret the motives and background of the other, "alien" partner to the contract, even though that person is not physically present in the consulting room. Of course, such interpretations should be employed only insofar as they illuminate who the *patient* is in light of those contracts and help him gain access to the pain – and its necessary grieving – that motivated their formation in the first place.

References

Abraham, N. and Torok, M. (1994). *The Shell and the Kernel: Renewals of Psychoanalysis*, Vol. I. (N. T. Rand, Trans. & Ed.). Chicago, IL: University of Chicago Press.

Beier, E. G. and Young, D. M. (1998). *The Silent Language of Psychotherapy*, Third Edition. New York: Aldine de Gruyter.

Berenstein, I. (2001). The link and the other. *International Journal of Psychoanalysis*, 82(1): 141–149.

Berenstein, I. (2009). Commentary: The concept of the link in couple and family psychoanalysis. In *International Review of Psychoanalysis of Couple and Family, No. 6*. International Association of Couple and Family Psychoanalysis, pp. 86–90.

Berenstein, I. (2012). *Vinculo* as a relationship between others. *Psychoanalytic Quarterly*, 81(3): 565–577.

Bolognini, S. (2004). Intrapsychic-interpsychic. *International Journal of Psychoanalysis*, 85(2): 337–358.

Broughton, J. L. (1999). *The Bodhidharma Anthology: The Earliest Records of Zen*. Berkeley, CA: University of California Press.

Davies, D. (2017). FBI profiler says linguistic work was pivotal in capture of Unabomber. Retrieved from www.npr.org/2017/08/22/545122205/fbi-profiler-says-linguistic-work-was-pivotal-in-capture-of-unabomber

Gabbard, G. O. (2012). Deconstructing vínculo. *Psychoanalytic Quarterly*, 81(3): 579–587.

Kaës, R. (1993). *Le Groupe et le Sujet du Groupe*. Paris: Dunod.

Kaës, R. (1995). L'exigence de travail imposée à la psyché par la subjectivité de l'objet. *Revue Belge de Psychanalyse*, 27: 1–23.

Kaës, R. (1998). L'intersubjectivité: Un fondement de la vie psychique. Repères dans la pensée de Piera Aulagnier. *Topique*, 64: 45–73.

Kaës, R. (2007). *Linking, Alliances, and Shared Space: Groups and the Psychoanalyst* (A. Weller, Trans.). London: International Psychoanalytical Association.

Kirshner, L. A. (2006). The work of Rene Kaës: Intersubjective transmission in families, groups, and culture. *Journal of the American Psychoanalytic Association*, 54(3): 1005–1013.

Lemma, A. and Target, M. (2011). *Brief Dynamic Interpersonal Therapy: A Clinician's Guide*. Oxford: Oxford University Press.

Losso, R., de Setton, L. S. and Scharff, D. E. (2017). *The Linked Self in Psychoanalysis: The Pioneering Work of Enrique Pichon Riviere*. London: Karnac.

Lyons-Ruth, K. (1999). The two-person unconscious. *Psychoanalytic Inquiry*, 19(4): 576–617.

Poulton, J. L. (2013). *Object Relations and Relationality in Couple Therapy*. Lanham, MD: Jason Aronson.

Puget, J. (2006). The use of the past and the present in the clinical setting. *International Journal of Psychoanalysis*, 87: 1691–1707.

Scharff, D. (2009). The concept of the link in couple and family psychoanalysis: Introduction. In *International Review of Psychoanalysis of Couple and Family, No. 6*. International Association of Couple and Family Psychoanalysis, pp. 68–85.

Stern, D. N. (1995). *The Motherhood Constellation*. New York: Basic Books.

Stern, D. N., Sander, L. W., Nahum, J. P., Harrison, A. M., Lyons-Ruth, K., Morgan, A. C., Bruschweilerstern, N. and Tronick, E. Z. (1998). Non-interpretive mechanisms in psychoanalytic therapy: The 'Something More' than interpretation. *International Journal of Psychoanalysis*, 79: 903–921.

Thomä, H. and Kächele, H. (1992). *Psychoanalytic Practice: 2-Clinical Studies*. Berlin, Heidelberg: Springer-Verlag, pp. 1–518.

Trevarthen, C. (1993). Brain, science and the human spirit. In J. B. Ashbrook et al. (Eds.), *Brain, Culture and the Human Spirit*. Lanham, MD: University Press of America, pp. 129–181.

3 Dreaming up, re-finding, and grieving lost objects

A case study

Carl Bagnini

This chapter describes a discovery process that fostered a change in the treatment of a very difficult case. Dream work on the therapist's part occurred at a crucial juncture of the treatment that transformed a difficult impasse into a creative encounter.

When the therapist dreams during analytic treatment, the dream has a dual function: the patient that is blocked prefers to remain asleep (unconscious), while the treatment situation stirs powerful countertransference images in the therapist's unconscious, whose dream can uncover subjective truths (evidence) crucial to opening up a new pathway for grieving lost objects in cases of trauma.

Theory and the evolution of technique in challenging cases

Contemporary psychoanalytic theory has expanded the study of internal and external objects and recognized that object relations are fluctuating ordinary relational phenomena occurring between therapist and patient. Traditional thinking had focused mainly on the object relations of the patient, with the therapist's position one of relative abstinence or neutrality. The material considered most relevant to therapeutic process consisted of the patient's utterances, dreams, associations, and transferences. As long as the therapist reflected on his or her countertransference as the product of and not the cause of patient transferences, patient-centered interpretations allowed the therapist a semblance of detached and benign objectivity. In this approach, patient personal history was the hidden treasure to be *mined* by the ready *mind* of the therapist.

The evolutionary world of psychoanalysis has expanded the study of object relations to the field of multiple psyches. Relational meanings of enactments, mental process, and attachment issues recast object relations as a system with new paradigms for treatment of deeply disturbed, dissociative, or otherwise stuck patients. We re-frame the frame in search of technical options with the most difficult cases. One of these options is to resist the temptation to quickly jump into transference interpretations before bearing the unknown and suffering with the unmetabolized beta elements of traumatic exposure. How do our psyches bear the experience of pain associated with patient trauma, and how does *our* traumatic past become the pathway for finding a transformative potential?

While we do not yet have sufficient research to empirically compare psychoanalytic models, we can study and consider what occurs that makes a difference one case at a time. In practice we cling to a preferred approach, while undergoing a seismic tilt that shakes our beliefs in what we are doing when reaching a limit in holding and containment. In the undertow of becoming personally disturbed, a discovery surfaces that makes a difference in the clinical situation. Was the change a product of theory, intuition, a mistake, or catastrophic acting out? Or was there a co-constructed image, perception, bodily sensation, thought, or intuition that created a new "gestalt"? Such a gestalt of complex properties and emotions has a re-organizing effect on the relationship, adding new meanings for use.

In the case presentation that follows I feature the importance of therapist's dreaming for retrieving and grieving lost objects as central to therapeutic progress. The dreamscape offers pathways to their access, but the process of discovery is arduous, personally upsetting, and indirectly discovered. In David E. Scharff's well-crafted book *Re-finding the Object and Reclaiming the Self* (1992), we are treated to a relational exploration of discovery and loss by examining what lies between and within ourselves and our patients in individual, couple, and family psychotherapy and psychoanalysis. In such explorations we are asked to probe the mutual shaping of patient and therapist object relations, in order to ground ourselves in a parallel process of discovering and grieving lost objects. I conjecture that we fall prey to, ignore, and escape opportunities and defend against affects that are central to retrieving lost objects.

Our historicized vulnerabilities interfere at first with re-finding our personal traumas, and locating patient defenses that parallel our unconscious fears and partially metabolized personal histories in avoiding theirs. We collude in having similar avoidances that require attentiveness and a willingness to suffer through "not knowing" (Bion, 1974). Gradually, if we are able to summon the courage and persist in locating the uncanny in us, a transformative potential can result that enhances the therapeutic relationship.

As we can see, the I-thou has grown to the I-thou-and-them – the unconscious relational others in the setting that make object relations more complex than we might be comfortable with. Evolving theory prompts the central question: Whose object relations are the focus of treatment? Relational models focus less on patient autonomy and more on the intersubjective matrix of the treatment dyad. While acknowledging that patient and therapist are individuals, the technical issues for relational analysts involve what to work on within a "co-constructed" environment. In current practice, therapists from other schools, including contemporary Freudians, modern Kleinians, ego psychologists, self-psychologists, Bionians, and others, variously conceptualize the individual mind as connected to a larger psychic world or field.

Let us now apply these observations to practice. When a therapist dreams during a treatment, this is a phenomenological event and requires a generous consideration of the multiple effects of interactive elements occurring between treatment participants. Dreaming can increase awareness in a therapist whose patient remains deeply unaware. When patient and therapist are locked into concrete transactions, the therapist can experience a "near" psychic death exposure; it is the impasse that forecloses availability for working in the symbolic realm. The therapist's dream can be influenced by the patient's ruthless shutting down of the therapist's emotional range, by numbing and repetition. Can we reduce the therapist's dream to a countertransference enactment, traceable to the therapist's all-too-willing emotional receptivity? Or might the dream function as a healing or contact point with self-objects for the therapist's personal benefit? Are we permitted to gain narcissistic supplies from our work?

What meaning, if any, does this all have with respect to the way I relate as a clinician and person? Although I respond to the existentialist in me, such a response privileges the here-and-now experience of patient-therapist encounters. I am deeply affected by various ways the therapeutic comes into being from surprises, mistakes, dreams, and associated somatic and painful stuck-ness. The psyche-soma of the therapist-patient relationship is an important dimension of the treatment.

In clinical practice we discover a unique unconscious sharing of mutually resonating self-parts, resulting in an expanded conceptualization of treatment, in which the contextual make up of human interaction is more important than patient internalizations alone. In this interface, there is an opportunity to be in touch with therapist and patient internal object worlds as they interact. These interactions produce a more inclusive, if not complete, experience. Exposure to each other's humanity in here-and-now relating has a profound impact on psychological process and outcome. Objects and part-objects press into the relationship, seek expression and then recognition. If they are not available in the patient's consciousness, they emerge in the therapist's subjective associations, crazy thoughts, dreams, and psychosomatic reactions in or between sessions.

Case studies are one means to empirically determine whether clinical theory works in practice. I have found that in certain clinical situations, we can draw inspiration and technical assistance from a flexible partaking from other models, in order to address particular difficulties when feeling limited in moving the treatment forward. Once we identify gaps in our own theory or technique, we can borrow from other models. Altering our analytic approach comes from practice over time; we are not the same therapist now as we were during or soon after completing training. Learning always implies change and a degree of suffering.

I want to turn to one of Bion's contributions to practice that assisted me in the case I describe later in this essay. The specific clinical idea is that patients express meanings without emotions and emotions without meanings (Bion, 1965, p. 183). The density of the patient-therapist exchanges becomes concrete, with fluctuations between two types of disturbances that reduce analytic work. Co-generated problems occur, as the field becomes laden with action-discharge *or* linguistic paralysis. The patient's symbols are conscious but have no transforming value; their emotions erupt without thought. Are we reduced to "pruners," reducing the patient's options out of sadistic reactivity, when caught up in our defenses against their ruthlessness (Bolognini, 2006, p. 114) or to being "dreamers," connoting a capacity to play? Our fantasies must remain hidden until something ripens, and if discovered and communicated. Then unrepresented objects may emerge and become newly represented.

I now explore a case that illustrates how an expanded cast of shadowy characters fostered dream work and tapped into unrepressed, unforgotten meanings that had not been thought by the patient or myself. The process of discovery caused turbulence. A seismic shift occurred first in the therapist and then in the patient as new meanings came to have an impact. I describe the emergence of the therapist's dream and how it opened a new space for moving the work forward. Self-discovery came with the therapist's dream work that accessed traumatic elements in both patient and therapist, freeing up the therapist to gain access to the patient's childhood trauma.

The case of Lanie

I am in my office with Lanie, 40, married, smart, and a beautiful, tall, blond former model, mother of two boys, 3 and 5. Very high strung, volatile, and disturbed, Lanie has been with me for two years in twice-a-week therapy. Her fluctuating moods and taste for marijuana and alcohol are my constant concern. Her difficult history involves anorexia-bulimia, beginning in her teens, then under control during her first pregnancy after in-patient treatment, and a masochistic attachment to a depressed, forced-into-retirement, and once very capable surgeon father, long divorced from mother, compulsively involved with two women. The women presumably do not know of the other lover.

Lanie has two brothers, one older, the other younger, each by two years. Younger brother is long-term dependent on father for financial survival and is a pot and cocaine user, unemployed and very volatile. Lanie tries to help by listening to him and ignoring his attacks on her "well-to-do life." Older brother is easier to talk to but blames father for everything wrong in his life. He loses jobs, cannot get along with bosses, and was estranged from father for four years after father left mother for another woman when Lanie was 18. Lanie is the "glue," as she puts it. Mother is the only family member in the nuclear group that all of the siblings have contact with. Mother is reported to be intellectual and cannot make decisions without the input of her second husband, a nice man who, unlike Lanie's father, takes care of mother. Mother was an elementary schoolteacher, retired, and has been remarried since Lanie was 25. Lanie has a cordial relationship with the stepfather. As she puts it: "As long as mother is happy I'm okay." Another issue with mother is that Lanie could never feel close to her, due to mother's aloofness and intellectualized attitude. In this sense Lanie feels quite deprived and has sought out her philandering father, to whom she often gives more than she receives.

We have been working with Lanie's many issues. An interior designer, she is terrified of getting work because she will be unable to deliver an adequate job or on time due to a lack of confidence. Since treatment began she has taken on a few jobs and done well, but she continues to undermine her talent. She is bored at home as a full-time mother. She has a few women friends who drink and smoke pot every afternoon, between 3 and 5 a.m. before their husbands return home from work. Lanie reports pot helps her zone out, with less anxiety about her life, which seems boring and unproductive. She used to live in the city and partied regularly, drinking and smoking pot in the glitzy world of fashion modeling, with her then boyfriend, now husband of seven years. He works in his family business for less money than he is worth.

Three years ago I saw them as a couple during their second pregnancy for six months before their child was born. They were fighting over the unplanned second pregnancy, blaming each other, while both knowing they were having unprotected sex. They admitted that neither paid attention to the consequences. The couple had moved to town after the birth of their first son, and Lanie had not adapted, preferring the fast-lane life of New York. Lanie is a borderline personality, volatile, depressive, self-indulgent, masochistic in family relations with male members, and lacking in boundary setting. She regularly gets high with girl friends when the children are playing in other rooms with the babysitter in charge. She has more conscious awareness lately that the pot is capable of affecting the children. She doesn't pass out but needs it for stimulation and says it prevents depression at the end of the day. She uses pot to be alert when her husband comes home. She reports the pot is a reward for being able to do the chores. There is no evidence of child neglect or overt aggression with the children. Her psychiatrist is trying Naltrexone 50 mg to reduce and structure alcohol consumption and as a substitute for rehabilitation, AA, or other treatments that would require exposure to addiction environments. Lanie refuses the other options out of shame. She cries when we discuss other approaches should the medication not work. She was drinking less wine by taking the medication, saying she has to drink for the medication to be effective. She also takes Xanax, Klonopin, and Prozac to stabilize her.

Recently (after two months) she is drinking more again, mostly wine at dinner that helps her relax, while insisting that Naltrexone can take six months to be effective. I believe this is pure rationalization, and I am expecting failure because Lanie is denying the extent of the dependency. Her husband is getting more upset with her. They still drink together, although he does not get incapacitated.

The marriage was based on early adolescent sexual excitement and partying, a mutual addictive fixation with youthful boundary testing, and later an adjustment to family life in suburbia, which brought responsibilities for children with Lanie hemmed in to a small-town life, isolation, and no career. The couple bickers over money, child rearing (she feels he's the calmer parent but dictates how she should do better), and extended family (Lanie cannot stand one of his sisters, whom he is close to. They gang up on her when they drink, pointing out Lanie's faults.).

Lanie appears for sessions dressed in tight stretch pants and loosely layered tops that move when she shifts in her chair. She is well groomed and uses makeup and has not come to sessions either high or sedated. She relates to me as safe to talk to, is often not sure where to begin, and at other times is worked up over extended family relations, her lack of happiness, and her inability to find her way in life.

Course of treatment

The first treatment was couple therapy for six month that stabilized the couple. They made adjustments in their expectations of each other after a period of angry blaming over the pregnancy, which we traced to insecurities and fears about taking on responsibilities for the changes.

Lanie called two years later for individual therapy, with symptoms of anxiety, depression, and malaise about life passing her by, with further disillusionment about marriage and motherhood. While she professed love for her husband and two boys, she claimed her husband's job gave his life meaning, while she missed city life. Marijuana and alcohol were always part of her life, and occasional blackouts had occurred in the city as well as in the suburbs, but she insisted it was when her husband became more worried that she had decided to try therapy. She feels responsible for her brothers' and father's dysfunctional life and relationships, but it is all she has to hold onto.

A major difficulty has been that Lanie appears to take in only shared observations or interpretive comments; these may come from my enlarging her narrative of early childhood neglect when I connect that to bad choices of exploitive males in late adolescence or college. She cries, then becomes very surprised to be feeling so strongly, as though her factual portrayal is more emotionally significant to me than to her. Then her retention of what occurred disappears and in the next session she asks me what we discussed in the previous one, saying that was probably important. I usually leave room for her to work with situations rather than coaching her. The going has been tough, given the powerful defenses against remembering and new emotional connections to the material and to me, the person responding in this unusual way. It is unlike any experience she has had before.

Gradually Lanie grew to tolerate my way of working, showing intellectual curiosity, but emotionally she hung onto what she knew – unprocessed, unmetabolized connections to her symptoms or personality difficulties. Attempts to discuss the overall influences of being tied to a masochistic-sadistic (I don't use these words) merry-go-round, family inheritance, and the way these keep her from detaching and individuating (including the addictive aspects) produces the same blockade of interest for a while. She questions my motives for bringing the patterns up but rationalizes that everything has to be what it is, lest her family be angry at her and she have no one. The neglect of herself and the self-defeating obligation to save others holds me hostage. I want to help her break free, but I feel I'm in the presence of a perversion of thought. The unrepressed fixed belief is that the bad is acceptable, and what is painful is the unmetabolized truth that I am holding. This is the scaffolding for undiscovered trauma.

A session

L. Not a good week. I spoke to my father yesterday *(begins to weep)* and he has Parkinson's you know. He was complaining about Eric again *(the younger, financially dependent brother)*. He got a DUI and wants my dad to take care of it.

TH. And the tears?

L. I don't know, it makes me sad that father is always pressured to bail out my brothers. He can't ever do enough to satisfy them.

TH. Are there other feelings or thoughts along with the tears when you listen to father?

L. I talk to my brothers and try to be understanding. I give them advice, asking them to give Dad a break. Eric turns on me, says that I should mind my own business, that Dad owes him. Dad wasn't around when we were kids. He was out working or having affairs *(I'm not sure if Lanie is reporting what Eric said or having a recollection)*. My father complains on the phone, then asks me out to dinner and I hear it all again. I tell him to take better care of himself, to enjoy life, but I know he isn't listening.

TH. And then?

L. *(Crying again more intensely.)* It's so frustrating I just want to run away, but he needs me. The alternating bimbos he brings to the house don't relate to me or the boys. Dad comes for an hour and disappears for weeks with the bimbos. He wants to talk about them to me because they want to marry him.

TH. You keep trying and nothing works. Let's consider the result! He runs away from your efforts to advise, then you want to run away from the rejection of your worried love for him. I wonder what's happening here between us!

L. What do you mean between us?

TH. Do you see a parallel?

L. Like I'm repeating the running away with you? That can't be. You're not like my father, you listen and try to help me.

TH. Lanie, the story you're re-telling has to do with you not feeling influential in your father's depressing life or your brother's, and you keep trying. There's no anger coming up when your efforts go in the toilet. I wonder if my efforts are following suit, because you are always sad and upset that your words don't improve things; I am feeling that here. Neither one of us is getting through to the other, so we're in the stuck place together.

L. No, Carl, that doesn't make sense. I am stuck, that's true, but I want your help. I don't want to give up drinking and pot though, which I believe you think would be good for me.

TH. And?

L. It would, but they give me peace and calm me down.

TH. Yes, that's all true. And you need their calming effects because that prevents other emotions from emerging that you are very fearful of – like anger. And yet you remain miserable and know it well.

L. I have to think about that. I can't follow that kind of logic.

TH. We have to stop now.

The therapist's dream followed this session:

> *I'm in a cab, driving through a vaguely familiar Brooklyn neighborhood. The driver is a Jamaican woman, lighthearted, with an infectious lyrical accent*

that makes me want to listen, not caring what she says because the music of her voice is so enthralling. In the dream, I'm much younger, in my early 30s, having worked in mostly minority neighborhoods, one in particular in which I was the only Caucasian social worker/child therapist. As is the local custom, the cab stops to pick up additional passengers while taking me on my journey to – I have no idea where. Three children enter the cab. The first is a black girl, about 9. A 7-year-old black girl pushes in behind; she doesn't look much like the first child, but I sense they are sisters, and after her, a white boy, about 12. To accommodate the three children, I shift as far to the right side of the back seat to make room. Being white, I am partly apprehensive I am going to have my wallet stolen by three hungry children. The driver is quiet. The girl closest to me says: "Do you have a father?" I reply, "I did, but he died a long time ago." She gazes left at the younger girl, pensive, leans closer to me, head almost touching my shoulder. "Lucy has no father, and she cries a lot, but I can deal." She speaks in a detached intellectual tone, then puts her head on my shoulder and begins weeping deeply.

I sit silently, quietly weeping, trying not to disturb her, and gently put my left arm around her shoulder. We are still now, both quiet, emotionally connected in grief, strangers in a cab, coming from and traveling together but in different directions. As she pulls over, the Jamaican cab driver, with her upbeat, musical voice, announces, "We're here." The dream ends.

Discussion

My dream suggests a powerful merged unconscious grief experience with Lanie, signaled by means of the cab ride with the three children. The eldest, a girl, nine, conveys her sister's father loss, after which she seeks comfort from me. My initial fear of having my wallet stolen by the hungry children connects to the fear that Lanie is depleting me, robbing me of my analytic resourcefulness. Lanie's primary family represents the core traumatic exposures of Lanie to resourceless dependency, which she projects onto me. The nine-year-old's intellectual telling of father loss reminds me of Lanie's mother, who intellectualizes most emotions, while relying extensively on a man to make her decisions. However, the nine-year-old girl transitions to weeping deeply, representing my conscious wish for Lanie, who I believe needs an emotional breakdown to retrieve lost objects. I am the shoulder she weeps on. While weeping myself, we share father loss, quietly, without conversation. The driver and the location (Brooklyn) are familiar figures from my own childhood. I imagine the driver is the *arms-around* Winnicottian figure, one that makes for a tight back seat but provides a sing-song container for a chance encounter on a journey that will takes us passengers to different destinations. The 12-year-old silent white boy represents me at that age, observing and fearful of experiencing female losses of fathers – a parallel tragic loss I could not share with the females in my family of origin.

The dream, therefore, represents a bridgeable moment between us as a therapy pair, at a time when Lanie's clinging to a life of numbness, isolation, and sacrifice is depleting my capacity to feel I am meaningful to her. In the sessions, we share the experience of trying and failing to engage, each feeling isolated and lost. I feel rejected and inadequate because my words fail to touch her, while she insists she needs me. Lanie strives but cannot rescue anyone, especially herself. Parts of myself and parts of Lanie's self are joined: Lanie insists she wants my help, a belief she relies on masochistically when relating to her own nuclear family that uses her. I feel used in a similar way: we talk, but she promptly forgets. I reflect on how I am engaging. My approach has been to link fears of her repressed aggression to her suffering and her escape into numbness through pot and alcohol. I am not getting to the traumatic elements in her life, however, or the depressed aspects she denies in favor of boredom.

Next session later that week

I'm feeling the dream's effects as I wait for the session to begin. I'm sad and burdened.

L. We were in an important place, right? Do you remember where we were last time *(embarrassed and blushing)*?

TH. What's it feeling like now, not being able to remember?

L. I don't know. It was very emotional, I think.

TH. I want to shift the subject. Can you recall what it was like between 3 p.m. and 5 p.m. weekdays as a child with Mom and Dad at work? *(The hours 3 to 5 p.m. surfaced in relation to the hours Lanie and her friends regularly partied. The numbing and the hours somehow resonated in me as having potential to shut out traumatic memories.)*

L. *(Sits forward and grips the sides of the chair.)* Nothing happened. My brothers and I carpooled with the neighbor's kids and their nanny, Felicia.

TH. *(I don't know why I shifted, but I am going with it because of the dream.)* And when you got home?

L. I did homework and had a snack.

TH. *(Feels intense and scary here.)* And your brothers? They were there?

L. No, I can't seem to find them. Maybe they were outside playing. *(Becoming increasingly uncomfortable, staring at me leaning forward.)* My brothers were playing. . . . *(Suddenly begins to sob! Covers her face with both hands.)* I told them to play inside, it was getting dark. I wanted to be included. Peter *(older)* said: "You're not my mother," and he and Eric were mad at me. I was scared when Peter got mad because he threw things, and my mother couldn't control him. I am feeling something bad happened.

(Lanie squeezes her legs together and turns away but keeps talking.) We played a game Peter said we could play together. He called it Explorer.

TH. Lanie, I'm here with you. How old were you at the time?

L. I was eight. Peter was big! He hurt me! I did what he said. He told me to undress, but he didn't. He said he got the first turn. Then he *(more sobbing but talking)* . . . pushed his finger inside me and in my backside too, and it hurt and he made Eric watch. He made me touch his penis. He said it felt good. . . . Should I tell you everything?

TH. Tell me what you've been holding inside all these years. And if you don't feel safe we can stop.

L. He was laughing. It hurt and he pushed harder. He wanted to use a wooden kitchen spoon, but Eric cried, so Peter put it away. I got dressed and ran to my room and cried. *(Lanie is crying, but I sense some relief because she can run to her room.)* I can't say anymore. It's terrible. My brother did this, and then I try to help him all these years. *(Lanie is crying, looking at me with sorrowful eyes)*.

L. Is this supposed to help me, Carl?

TH. You seem angry with me now because we released a terrible memory. The anger at Peter for causing you pain was never expressed because of fear. We need to consider where the anger belongs. How about your parents?

L. I never told anyone. I tried to forget.

TH. And you became the dutiful child obligated to keep men from losing control or falling apart.

End of session.

Discussion and conclusion

In this session, Lanie was able to connect emotionally to the therapist by means of the shift to his association that seemed to appear out of nowhere. The affect that was revealed had been blocked throughout Lanie's life. The issue of mourning losses might have been accomplished gradually if Lanie had felt safe enough to remember how the losses occurred: Her brothers' sadism, Lanie's shame, terror, loneliness, being left unprotected, secrecy, lack of safety and mistrust – all missing fundamental requirements for healthy development.

The emergence of the therapist's dream at a critical point in treatment expanded the possibilities in a stuck situation. Theory about treatment expands the study of therapist-patient object relations when there is a blurring of boundaries that occurs with deeply wounded patients that challenges analytic neutrality. Objectivity becomes useless and potentially results in the therapist's defensive counter-resistance. A patient's dream in a "waking" state within the holding environment may be too close to annihilative anxieties, because it has the potential to elicit the panic of going "mad." Because of the defenses that numb madness, a patient's life has been lived without concern for consequences. The patient in this case was less re-traumatized because she did not know that the therapist, as proxy and guardian of the patient's waking and sleeping life, had a co-created dream that led to an opportunity to move beyond the impasse and salvage treatment. The location and retrieving of lost objects and the opportunity to mourn in instances like this can aid the creation and application of a therapist's dream.

References

Bion, W. R. (1965). *Transformations: Change from Learning to Growth*. London: Heinemann.

Bion, W. R. (1974). *Experiences in Groups and Other Papers*. London. Tavistock.

Bolognini, S. (2006). *Like Wind, Like Wave: Fables from the Land of the Repressed*. New York: Other Press.

Scharff, D. E. (1992). *Re-Finding the Object and Reclaiming the Self*. Northvale, NJ: Jason Aronson.

4 Creating a new relationship in child analysis

Revisiting theoretical ideas of developmental and transference objects

Caroline Sehon

Introduction

I had the privilege to meet "Ella" when she was four years nine months old. An only child, Ella was born to parents in their late 30s who wrestled for several years about whether to conceive, frightened of recapitulating their own traumatic family histories. The mother worked from home as an entrepreneur of a small start-up company, and the father traveled often as a salesman.

Ella's parents consulted me at the recommendation of her preschool teacher. A bright, creative, and determined little girl, Ella was hampered by severe emotional, social, and academic delays. She was further challenged by a serious speech articulation problem – she became extremely frustrated and prone to meltdowns when people made clumsy efforts to decode her unrecognizable words. Her mother reported that Ella had a "latching problem" at birth, such that "I didn't produce enough milk, and she didn't naturally take milk." At one week of life, breastfeeding was quickly halted when her mother noticed that "the nurses were shoving the nipple into her mouth and it was really invasive." Subsequently, Ella expressed strong food preferences and resistance to eating solids. Apparently unable to sense her need to relieve her full bladder or bowel, she also faced the occasional embarrassment of enuretic or encopretic episodes.

At the start of our journey, Ella suffered also with profound separation anxiety, especially from her mother. She was frequently required to play alone when her mother teleworked from home and conducted daily business calls in private. Time and time again, she tried to enter her mother's office, only to be ushered away. Although her mother was otherwise involved in her life, these moments occurred consistently, leaving Ella feeling dropped. Similarly, her father was absent for long workdays or on travel; upon his reentry, he was often asleep or too tired to play with her. A similar dynamic therefore unfolded between Ella and each parent in which she would meet a seemingly present parent who was actually unavailable. These contrasting settings set the stage, in my view, for anxiety within Ella, between Ella and her parents, and between Ella and me in the transference surrounding recurrent fears of separation and rejection on one hand and her desperate longing for closeness and merger on the other.

Many parents feel paralyzed about crossing the therapeutic threshold because of guilt about their contributions to their child's problems. Ella's parents were no exception. They openly expressed deep pain at having to revisit their own sense of childhood trauma and at exposing their misgivings about their perceived parenting failures. Yet they were able to secure a strong therapeutic alliance with me, and they became unwaveringly devoted to Ella's treatment.

Favorable results were achieved with a one-year course of twice-weekly analytic therapy, once-weekly parent work, and speech therapy (provisioned privately), but Ella still had fierce trouble handling her intense feelings, conflicts, and separation anxieties and representing her aggressive feelings and affectionate longings through play or words. The parents therefore accepted my offer of a four-times-weekly analysis along with once-weekly parent work.

This essay focuses specifically on Ella's use of various therapeutic "objects" at successive and ever-deepening moments along the analytic journey. Over the course of the analysis, she and I embarked upon a *spiral process* (Scharff, Losso and Setton, 2017) in which Ella became gradually more capable of employing me as a *transference object* and relatively less as a *developmental object* (Neely, 2020, in press). In one sense, therapeutic action is regarded as occurring within an analytic field, in which the heart of the action occurs within the setting of *el vinculo* or "links" that represent numerous relational patterns, affects, transference and countertransference manifestations, and traumatic experiences transmitted both intergenerationally and within the here-and-now of the child's family and surrounding communities (Scharff and Scharff, 2011; Sehon, 2013).

The emerging development of transference and countertransference requires the child to find and employ the analyst as a *transference object* in progressive ways. In a complementary manner, it is necessary for the analyst to be used and created by the child as a *transference object* and for the analyst to welcome the child patient as a "countertransference object." This interpenetration of subject and object within the shared mind of the analytic pair takes time and patience before the analyst can glean hints of the transference. Then, proper tact and timing are needed for the analyst to offer a transference interpretation as a hypothesis, delivered into the displacement of the play or directly to the child. Many factors determine a child's capacity to use such transference interpretations, not the least of which is the child's developmental readiness. If all goes well, the analytic couple will leverage such work in the transference-countertransference field to collaborate on behalf of the child resolving her conflicts and advancing her development.

But how would the child patient make optimal use of the analyst as a *transference object* if she were severely developmentally delayed and subject to ongoing family strain or traumatic *links*? The term "developmental object" was coined by Tähkä to describe the analyst's capacity to identify the patient's developmental needs and potentials and to facilitate a transformation in the child's difficulties as they will be repeated within the analytic relationship (Tähkä, 1993). This construct was subsequently elaborated by Anne Hurry, Jill Miller, Carla Neely, and others to capture something of the deeply moving and often memorable moments of intimate interaction between the child and the analyst that support the child's development. When the analyst is receptive to being found and used by the child as a *developmental object*, she resonates with those developmental needs transmitted by the child through play or words.

Winnicott described the analyst as functioning in this context as the *environment mother*, hopefully as a "good-enough mother (parent)" (Winnicott, 1965). David E. Scharff and Jill Savege Scharff elaborated on Winnicott's notion by introducing the term "contextual transference" to represent the child's experience of the analyst and the setting as either safe and welcoming – expressed as a *positive contextual transference* – or threatening and rejecting when it manifests as a *negative contextual transference* (Scharff and Scharff, 1998). Usually both elements co-occur, but the hope is that the positive contextual dimension will supersede the negative aspects. In this way, a sturdy therapeutic alliance forms between the child and the analyst, and in turn, the child marshals the analyst's capacity to serve as a *developmental object.*

Furthermore, the Scharffs conceptualized the *focused transference* as analogous to Winnicott's *object mother* and described the patient's use of the therapist as an object upon whom to project the exciting and rejecting object relationships (or aggressive and libidinal object relations). Through the analyst's availability as a *developmental object*, a *focused transference* eventually emerges in the form of a veritable transference neurosis when the child finds and creates the analyst as a *transference object* (Chused, 1988; Scharff and Scharff, 1998).

The concepts of the *developmental object* and the *transference object* are distinguishable from each other, yet they inherently operate at one and the same time. The use of one facilitates the improved use of the other. The clinical case material that follows provide examples to illustrate Ella's eager search for a *developmental object* to foster her progressive movement through her developmental impasse within the arms-around holding of the therapeutic relationship. As the analysis progressed, the analyst was able to make more transference interpretations both in the displacement and directly, in ways that were possible only because of the child's development and the growth of the analytic partnership. Over time, Ella's predominant use of the analyst as a *developmental object* receded, thus paving the way for the *transference object to take center stage.*

Description of child and setting

Ella was a pretty, highly intelligent, creative, inquisitive, engaging, and energetic little girl. At times, she appeared friendly and excited to meet with me, but on the turn of a dime she could become tearful, dramatic, angry, and commanding, or solemn, sad, and in retreat. From the beginning, she demonstrated a high capacity for symbolic play and prided herself on being able to distinguish between pretend play and reality. She had an innovative ability to create props at will – for example, she created an imaginative garden scene by lifting up toy flowers to combine with tree silhouettes that cast a shadow on the upper wall of my office.

At the start of our work, Ella often wore leggings under an oversized dress. Her hair was often uncombed as if she had just come running in from a storm; her straggly bangs often obscured her vision and kept me from seeing her eyes. Gradually her attire shifted to wearing more fitted skirts and pants, paired with decorative t-shirts that displayed hearts, ice cream cones, and various Disney characters. As the analysis progressed, she showed a more consistently pulled-together look, as signaled by her braided or neatly combed hair, pulled back from her face, and often adorned with colorful hair bands or barrettes.

Ella always impressed me as having the capacity to engage collaboratively. She seemed to enjoy the close-in attentiveness and understanding. Curious to listen and consider the meaning of my interpretative comments, she often demonstrated a short while thereafter that she had taken onboard a word or an idea from an earlier moment together. She was not at all shy to communicate her strong feelings, including her upset and her criticism of me. Sometimes, Ella was quick to take on the role of a pretend schoolteacher who told me the rules or scolded me for my "misbehaviors." For example, she would say sternly: "Shh! Shh! Leave me alone!" Or she would alternate a play sequence, one moment by working with me at the child table, then suddenly taking the toy characters to the floor where I could no longer see what she was doing or hear what she was saying.

Ella's communicative disturbances were a formidable hurdle for me to manage at the beginning of the therapy. At first, her words tumbled out, rapid-fire, in a jumbled, condensed manner. I found myself trying even harder to decipher her messages. I wondered: Was she beckoning me, or creating a barrier to what she had to say? Perhaps both hypotheses were true, as I reflected that she was probably expressing conflict for me both to hear and not to hear her. I suspected that my feelings of confusion and helplessness were at times reflective of her disorientation in a complex world that overwhelmed her. Fierce confrontations had developed with her mother whenever Ella grew frustrated by her mother's difficulty making sense of her words. Therefore, I refrained from having Ella repeat what she said and simply tried to immerse myself in the feeling of "not-knowing" (Bion, 1962) and in the profound symbolic richness of her play. Over time, I came to understand her words most of the time. Looking back, I think this situation resulted, in part, from an actual growth in her language ability (as noted objectively by the speech therapist and by her parents), from my learning to decode her "language" over time, and from her symptomatic relief as we slowly worked through some of her conflicts.

Ella's creativity and hunger for a relationship knew no bounds. She regarded each and every element of the physical setting as a potential vehicle through which to convey her conflicts and internal psychic life. From the get-go, she redesigned the office setting into an "open-floor" plan that included the sparsely furnished waiting room. One of the functions of this enlarged play space was to reveal her rejecting object relationship (Fairbairn, 1952). By claiming the waiting room as *her* private territory, in effect, she banished her mother from *her* space to symbolically retaliate against her mother, who turned her away from her business calls, or against her father, who traveled or retreated to bed. Once I realized that Ella was occupying the waiting room, in part, as a way to exclude her parents, I secured an alternate waiting room from one of my colleagues for the parents' use. In no uncertain terms, Ella was also asserting her agency and control in relation to me and the setting as *transference objects*.

Initially, the sessions took place entirely in the waiting room. Later, she moved to and fro between the office and the waiting room. As Ella conquered her separation anxieties and worked through various conflicts and traumas, she relied less on the waiting room, transitioned more easily from the waiting room into the office, and allowed me eventually to close the door for "our privacy." I provisioned Ella with her own box for her drawings that she chose to keep at the office, and I took a photographic record of drawings she wished to take home.

Vignettes over the course of the analysis

To illustrate Ella's use of diverse therapeutic objects, I selected several vignettes from the initial session and the early to middle phases of the analysis, between when she was four years nine months old until when she was six years four months old. I highlight how I understood my role in advancing Ella's development and the rationale for why I intervened in the way I did at particular *points of urgency* (Baranger, 1993).

Vignette no. 1 (our first encounter)

My first meeting with Ella, when she was four years nine months old, etched an indelible mark in my mind. I was drawn to her way of relating to me, to the office toys, and to the analytic setting as both *transference* and *developmental objects*. I felt her willful desire to be seen and known by me and her fierce determination to convey the troubled and resilient areas of her inner world. Although her words were sparse and her articulation distorted, her narrative was compelling nonetheless.

With eager anticipation, I expected to discover an involved mother-child pair given her extreme separation anxiety. On the contrary, Ella unhesitatingly parted from her mother and walked stoically into the office. A complex scene unfolded. Without making eye contact or uttering a word, she collapsed to the floor and examined the toys from a safe distance. I knelt next to her, watched, waited, and followed her lead. Hedging her bets, she glared at the toy animals and crawled on all fours, as if mimicking an animal in the wild facing a crowd of ominous predators that she would have to either fight or flee. Throughout the first 20 minutes, she remained mute. In tandem with her hypervigilant stance, I noticed ways that I felt gripped by this unusually dramatic entrée into our work together. She seemed to regard the toys as a potential danger. In contrast, she appeared to feel safe, as she crawled next to me on the floor, as if inviting me to join her as a co-investigator into this novel environment and into her inner world.

Then the atmosphere shifted to become soft and calm. Ever so slowly, she warmed to my offer to explore objects within her view. She tentatively reached out to pick up a tiny baby doll. I responded in a quiet, gentle, whispering voice: "Oh! A baby!" In turn, she picked up a miniature sleeping bag and then repeatedly tried to force a larger baby doll into the unyielding small space of the sleeping bag. When I commented, "Oh, the baby doesn't seem to fit in that small space," she persisted energetically until finally surrendering from fatigue. Although I uttered a few words, she held hers back as if to minimize the chance of feeling dropped by me. As I had learned that her garbled words often "fell on deaf ears," I suspected that she would need time before she could entrust me with her words. In resonance with her mute stance, I also felt lost for words amid intense feelings of curiosity and concern. A short while later, she picked up the wheelchair in the dollhouse and then, suddenly, a small girl doll fell over.

ANALYST: Oh!
ELLA: *(Uttering her very first words)*
She fell over!!
ANALYST: Oh! Ouch! Is she hurting?
ELLA: *(Emphatically)*
No!! She's okay.
ANALYST: Oh, maybe it hurt her, at first. We can pretend.
ELLA: *(Louder and insistently)*
No!! She's okay.
ANALYST: Oh, okay.
ELLA: *(She pretended to fly a butterfly and suddenly dropped it.)*
(Flatly, she said) It died.
ANALYST: Oh, it died! Oh, that's sad!
ELLA: *(She smiled and laughed.)*
ANALYST: Oh?! You're laughing, but the butterfly died.
ELLA: *(She picked up another butterfly on the bookcase and lifted it up in the air.)*
(With excitement) Look! Look! A purple butterfly!
ANALYST: Yes, it's so pretty.
ELLA: *(She pretended it was flying, stopped it in flight, and then looked at me while continuing to hold it airborne.)*
ANALYST: Oh! What's happening?!
ELLA: It's thinking.
ANALYST: *(I was utterly amazed by her remark and the sense that we had just taken a quantum leap forward.)*
Oh, okay! Let's give it time to think.

[There was a timeless quality to the atmosphere as she continued to hold the butterfly in the air, shifting her gaze back and forth between me and the butterfly. We both waited, looking together at the butterfly and at each other. I was fascinated by Ella's play. A short while later, I spoke softly, again with curiosity.]

I wonder what the butterfly is thinking. I'm going to ask the butterfly. What are you thinking, *Butterfly*?

ELLA: *(Gazing seriously at me)*
Are you pretending?

ANALYST: Yes, I'm pretending. We can do that together. . . .
(Near the end of the session, as I returned the dollhouse to its usual location, suddenly Ella pled her case.)

ELLA: I want you to keep all the same.

ANALYST: Okay, I will try hard to keep the toys in the same place.

* * * * *

In a certain sense, we can regard this first encounter as representing a fractal that foreshadows and summarizes the entire story of the analysis. What are the *anchor points* of this narrative (Bernardi, 2014)? Ella conveyed an image of a child who moved about the world as a baby, unable to support her weight as expected by her age and developmental stage. She made tireless efforts to push a baby doll into the "crawl space" of the toy sleeping bag, as if to convey her sense that earlier developmental needs had gone unheeded. She picked up a wheelchair, perhaps symbolically suggesting her need for holding and repair of her broken self. The first butterfly dropped to the floor and died, suggesting Ella's meltdowns when she became overwhelmed in the absence of holding and containment. Was she conveying her unconscious hope for a *second* chance, in which she and I would help her grow thinking capacity, just as the *second* butterfly could do? Defensively, she expressed an illusion of infantile omnipotence, declaring emphatically that the baby was numb to the pain of being "dropped." At the same time, she expressed the desire to find a "good-enough," accepting, new object relationship to afford her a sense of safety, where things are "(kept) all the same" and where thinking (and a mind) could develop at long last.

In summary, this first vignette spoke to her wish for a secure base and for her use of me as a *developmental object* that would allow her to unveil earlier selves that longed to speak and be heard. This inaugural scene displayed images of a split, *contextual transference* to me as both a benevolent and a malignant object. Although I was in role both as a *transference object* and as a *developmental object*, my hope at this stage was merely to take my first baby steps forward as Ella's analyst. I aimed to earn her trust as a *developmental object*, as someone who would listen to her, mirror her initial utterances, and encourage a gradually deepening conversation with me through play and language. On the basis of her early powerful impact on me that would eventually develop into a complex countertransference, I was beginning to form hypotheses for how Ella might discover and employ me as a *transference object*, as her internal mother, father, and other important attachment figures. In the meantime, I needed to remain in a state of suspended animation and of "not knowing" (Bion, 1962) and to enjoy the intrigue and mystery of the here-and-now with Ella.

Early phase of psychoanalytic therapy

Ella readily settled into the twice-weekly analytic therapy. At the start of each session, I usually discovered her at the child table in the waiting room, immersed in her drawing, while her mother read nearby. Ella conveyed her need for me to witness her first drawing of the day while we sat silently together in the waiting room. Sometimes she enjoyed commanding me to bring her markers from inside the office. I found this request to be particularly compelling given that she already had access to an identical set of markers in the waiting room. I surmised that Ella needed to use me as a *developmental object* in this way so as to create a symbolic bridge between the waiting room and my office. I thought she was partnering with me to bolster her nascent self-regulating function as she struggled to transition from her life at school, to her commute to my office with her mother, and finally to our play space.

Using me as a *transference object*, Ella kept me waiting at the start of sessions by demanding "Privacy! Privacy!" She insisted that I not look at or speak to her as she collected her thoughts and feelings represented through pictures or play. This resounding phrase, "Privacy! Privacy!," seemed highly precocious for a child of this age, and all the more so for Ella given her language delays. I wondered if she was repeating this command to re-enact a dynamic with me that echoed her mother's use of that phrase. At times, if I simply said, "Hmm," or, "I see many hearts on your drawing," she would say in a pseudo-adult voice, "Wait! I am working! . . . I need to do this! . . . I need my privacy!" Although she appeared anxious when her mother left, it was not unusual for Ella to later press up against the time boundaries at the end of the sessions so as to keep both her mother and me waiting.

In the early phase of our work, Ella spoke in a strident, demanding, urgent tone, lest I not take her seriously or question whether she was in charge. She would decide when she was ready to leave the waiting room, and she seemed pleased at being able to reject my invitation into the office. She hurled her directives like projectiles, putting me on notice to stay out of her play, regardless of whether I briefly commented or intervened in a careful and sensitive way. At times, she would yell, "Stop! Stop! My brain hurts!" or she would cry or collapse onto the floor. As she settled into the sessions, her affect usually became calmer and she could engage in symbolically rich play. She seemed to derive pleasure at making eye contact, at my tracking her play, and at our shared engagement that nonetheless emphasized her lead role. During this early phase, she occasionally allowed me to make brief comments about our interaction.

Although the transference became clearer over time, she often blocked me from making any direct transference interpretations. For example, she might say, "Now, now! Let's not talk about that right now!" Instead, I gathered the transference to me or made transference interpretations in the displacement, while serving primarily as a *developmental object*.

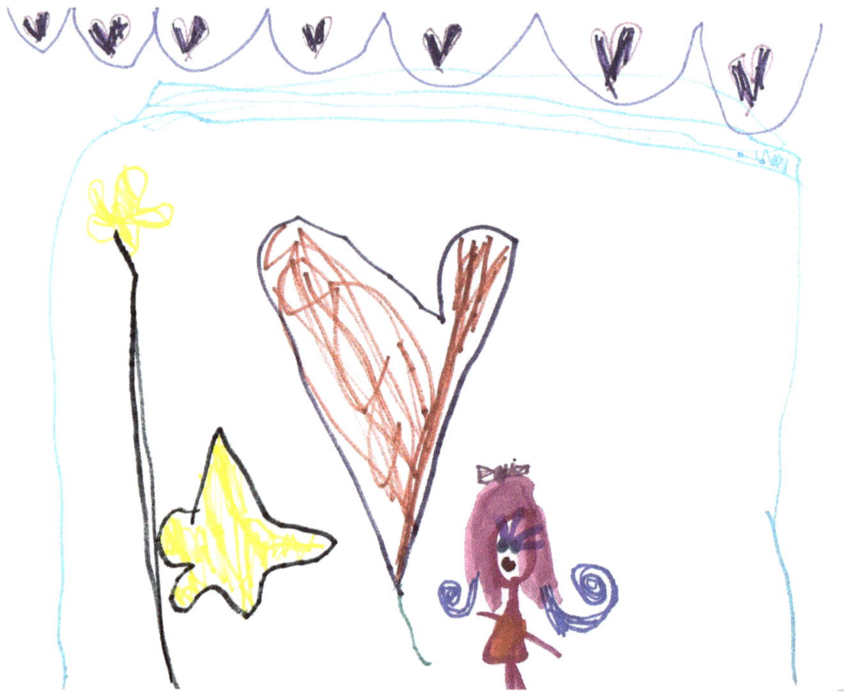

Figure 4.1 Baby

Early to middle phases of the psychoanalysis

Vignette no. 2

Although Ella showed no separation anxiety in the initial meeting, this quickly gave way to her becoming extremely anxious when her mother would depart. The parent work helped the mother hold firm as she assured Ella of her return 45 minutes later. During the first few months of the analysis, I often discovered a gripping image of Ella sobbing in the waiting room with her mother sitting nearby. This phenomenon initially surprised me given Ella's insistence that her mother not occupy the waiting room and given her frequent reluctance to leave the office at the end of the hour. Later I came to appreciate that this dramatic display of anxiety partly seemed aimed at reassuring her mother of her importance and value in Ella's mind.

After the mother departed, Ella often collapsed on the floor of the waiting room into a formless heap and soothed herself by twirling her fingers atop the white noise machine with my silent presence nearby. Or she would lean her spine against the legs of adjacent chairs as if to collect herself by means of a hard, *autistic object* (Tustin, 1980). Through these moments that lasted usually 10 or

15 minutes, I labored with feelings of helplessness as I witnessed her annihilation anxiety. As I discovered that my words caused her more distress, I learned that my quiet presence offered her the salve to recover more of her collaborative self.

On this occasion, it had been a few months since she had exhibited such extreme separation anxiety, so I was perplexed that we were revisiting this situation. As her mother got up to leave, Ella clung to her mother's leg and wailed and whined. The mother reported that Ella had just become extremely upset after getting water on her dress and that Ella's distress had escalated when the mother comforted her. Shortly thereafter, her mother left.

ELLA: *(Yelling loudly and angrily)* Privacy!! Privacy!!

ANALYST: Oh, okay. I'm going to sit here now. I will not look at you, Ella, to give you the privacy you are asking for. *(I was reminded of the gaze aversion to which infants resort as a way of self-soothing in the face of a depressed or overexciting object.)*

ELLA: *(A short while later, she slowly crawled down from the adult chair to her usual place at the child table in the waiting room and began drawing.)*
I don't want to talk! I need my privacy!

ANALYST: Yes, I'm going to draw here next to you. I'm not going to talk right now to give you your privacy.

For about ten minutes, we drew side by side. I noticed she would look up at me in a seemingly purposeful way as if communicating nonverbally that she valued my calm and quiet presence and my availability to speak or engage with her when she felt ready. I followed her lead and returned her gaze from time to time. She seemed to calm down further when our gaze met.

ANALYST: When you feel calmer, I would like to have a chat with you.

ELLA: I'm not calm. I need to draw until I'm calm.

ANALYST: Yes, drawing can sometimes help you feel calm when you're upset.

ELLA: *(Looking at me affectionately, she scribbled in the heart.)* Baby. Baby.

ANALYST: Baby.

ELLA: *(She completed the drawing, gathered herself, and looked up at me with self-composure.)*
Okay! I am ready now.

ANALYST: Okay. *(We entered the office together, and I closed the door to the waiting room behind us.)* . . .

As the session neared its end, she reverted to hurling "Privacy!" and tried to prolong the session rather than reunite with her mother. The following exchange captures a common pattern at this phase of our work.

ANALYST: It's time now for us to stop for today.

ELLA: No! I'm still working! Privacy! Privacy! *(She opened the door to glance at her mother and then slammed the door and remained with me. She repeated this sequence a few times while smiling and giggling.)*

ANALYST: Oh! You're in charge!

ELLA: *(She transformed into a calm and collected little girl and seemed interested in my comment.)*
I'm not in charge!! Why am I in charge?!

ANALYST: At the moment, you're in charge about when you will go out to see your mom.

ELLA: *(With mild pleasure, she repeated this sequence an additional few times, seemingly enjoying that she held the power and control. On the turn of a dime, as if commanding a Broadway performance, she looked at me, morphing into an extraordinarily pleasant child as if interested only in complying with my authority. In a charming way, she looked at me while wearing a half-smile, and asked in a coquettish voice)*
Can I leave now?

ANALYST: Yes.

After gently opening the door and leaving it slightly ajar, she reunited with her mother. In an unprecedented manner, she hurried back a few moments later, peeked inside the office, smiled at me, and then promptly slammed the door behind her. Effectively she had trapped me in the office. I was gripped by this unusual sequence that erupted beyond my control and by her crafty way of defying the time boundaries until *she* would emphatically decide when the session was over. Then I opened the door, looked at her attentively and with a partial smile, as a way of signaling that her aggression had not "killed me" off and of marking these moments that would need to be unpacked and understood on another day.

* * * * *

At the start of the session, Ella became unmoored when she accidentally wet her dress. I suspected she was angry at her mother for not protecting her from her own mishap. In all probability, her aggression disorganized and frightened her, especially given that her mother left shortly thereafter. Perhaps this sequence confirmed Ella's unconscious fear that her aggression could be "deadly." As I slowly became the recipient of Ella's anger, she found comfort in knowing that I would remain with her without retaliating and without leaving. In other words, Ella needed to use me and the setting as *developmental objects* to gather herself. Her fear and annihilation anxiety were at an all-time high, and her capacity for thinking was at an all-time low. It seemed to me that she could not use direct transference interpretations at moments when her sense of self was so fragile. Although I continued to listen to the transference, I aimed mainly to support her self-soothing through use of me as a *developmental object*.

This elaborately enacted narrative signaled also how Ella had used the temporal and physical dimensions of the setting as a proxy for me in role as a *transference object*. She seemed intent on my momentarily experiencing her hatred of the fact that I controlled the time boundaries. During these early days, her aggression came into the room mainly at such moments of separation, probably when she felt safe. In this exchange, there was no disputing that she had effectively used me as a *transference object*. I had become the internal mother. Ella thus marked a transformative moment in the analytic journey, signaling that she was now ready to work directly in the transference.

Vignette no. 3

This vignette marked another important shift in the work, as Ella seemed capable of using me more as a *transference object* than as a *developmental object*. At parent meetings, I had learned that Ella had become frightened by heated verbal altercations between her parents. During this phase of our work, Ella seemed to draw

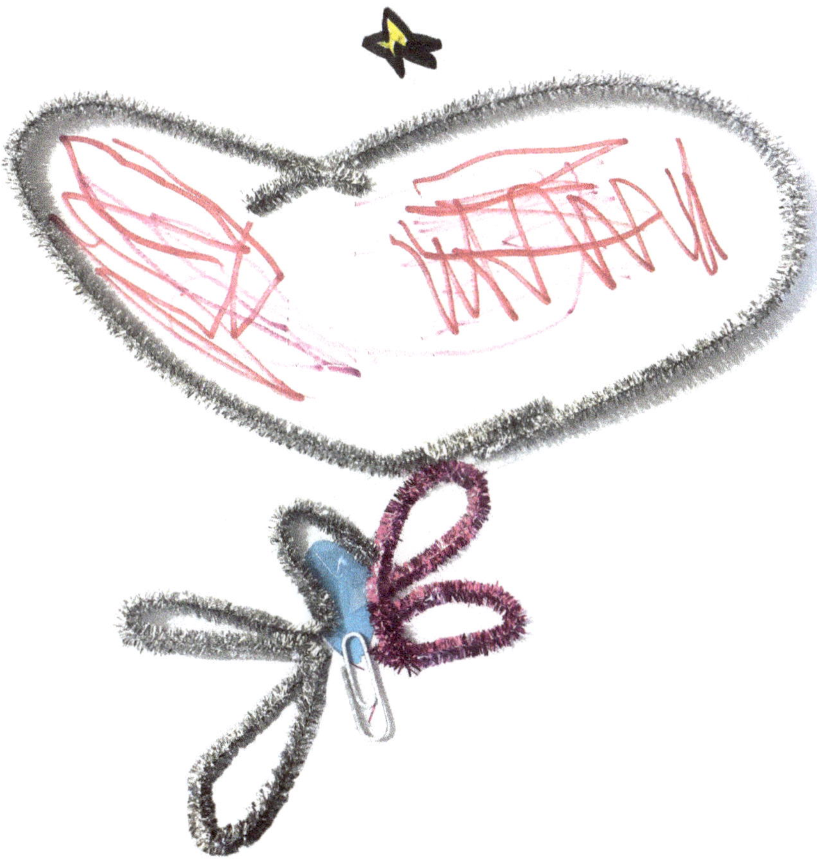

Figure 4.2 Flower petals

comfort from my welcoming her aggression toward me by "wearing the negative attributes," so she, in turn, could withstand her own aggression. We also had been working on her disappointment that I could not read her mind, which would have relieved her of having to verbalize her feelings and thoughts. That would have proved that I perfectly understood her. I suspected she longed to become at one with me as her *internal mother*, while she feared such intense closeness would threaten her sense of self. Over previous weeks, Ella and I had been working on distinguishing those times when she needed my assistance from moments when she could exercise her independence. Occasionally, she summoned the courage to express her helplessness and neediness by hurling a command for "Help!," albeit with an angry tone.

ELLA: *(She asked for help by asking me to place a silver pipe cleaner to form the petals of a flower without giving me specific instructions.)* *(sternly)* "No!! Not like that!"

ANALYST: Oh! I got that wrong! You seem upset with me.

ELLA: *(Immediately, she tried to do it in her own way but was terribly disappointed by the results.)*
Ughh!

ANALYST: Oh! Now you seem upset with yourself!

ELLA: *(She darted several feet away to take refuge under the child table.)*

ANALYST: Oh! You have leaped away, almost as if you are giving yourself a time out.

ELLA: *(From under the table, she faced me, and smiled. Then she reached for a light switch, turning it on and off repeatedly.)*
(Excitedly) Look!

ANALYST: Yes! I see the light is going on and off, on and off. One moment it is on, and the next moment it is off. That's like what happened here, one moment you're not upset, and another moment you are upset.

ELLA: *(In a sing-song voice, she made up the following song.)*

You're my best friend ever
You can be my best friend forever
You can be my best friend forever
I love to say
You are the best thing for me
I know you can be my best friend forever
So you can see
You're my best friend ever

* * * * *

On this occasion, Ella flew into a rage because I incorrectly shaped the flower petal. Then, she turned her aggression back on herself, after painfully realizing that she was unable to rely upon me as a mind reader. Her sense of pseudo-omnipotence began to crumble, and her aggression toward me threatened her sense of safety. She risked losing me as a *developmentally* "good-enough" *object*, only to feel in the hands of a negative *transference object* that could reject her by abandoning or turning against her. She exclaimed "Ughh!" in self-disgust, as if she had turned herself into a "bad object" in order to rescue me as a good mother in the transference (Fairbairn, 1952). Frightened, she sought refuge under the child table, as if the physical setting were a proxy for a positive *developmental object* that could reliably offer her safety and comfort.

By this point in the analysis, Ella was able to utilize the language and understanding I provided as a *container*, rather than relying principally upon me in more primitive ways. Ella's playful use of the light switch seemed to reflect her capacity to work in the transference. We could now engage in an elaborate narrative where distorted beliefs about herself and about me could be transformed (between "on" and "off"), rather than her simply holding both of us to a fixed position in which she was in charge and I was embattled. Near the end of the session, she gifted me with her song that celebrated our valued partnership and her creation of me as a "new object" with whom she had fallen in love and toward whom she could express rage without her world collapsing.

During this session, it seemed clear to me that she had found and used me as her *internal mother*. While I listened to the transference, it still felt premature for me to interpret her aggression as an attack upon her sense of neediness. Therefore, I continued primarily to serve as a *developmental object* by supporting her capacities to self-regulate; to assert her agency; to tolerate ambivalent feelings; and to grow her confidence in the analytic relationship. Nevertheless, the heat of the action still seemed more centered on her creating and using me as *a transference object*.

Vignette no. 4

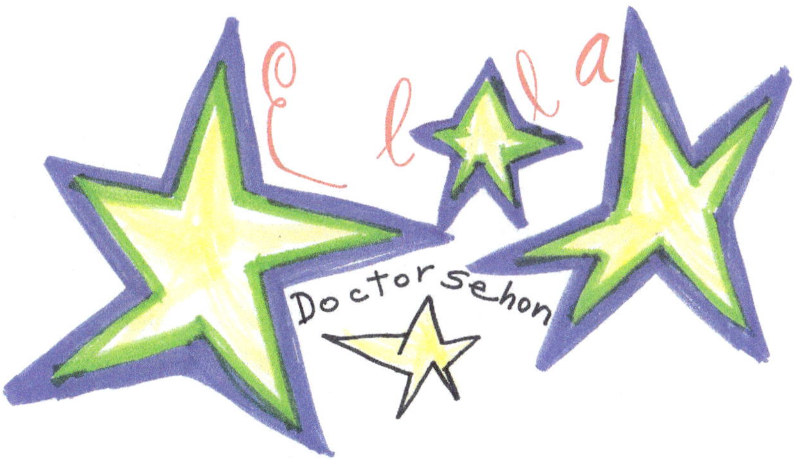

Figure 4.3a Constellation of stars

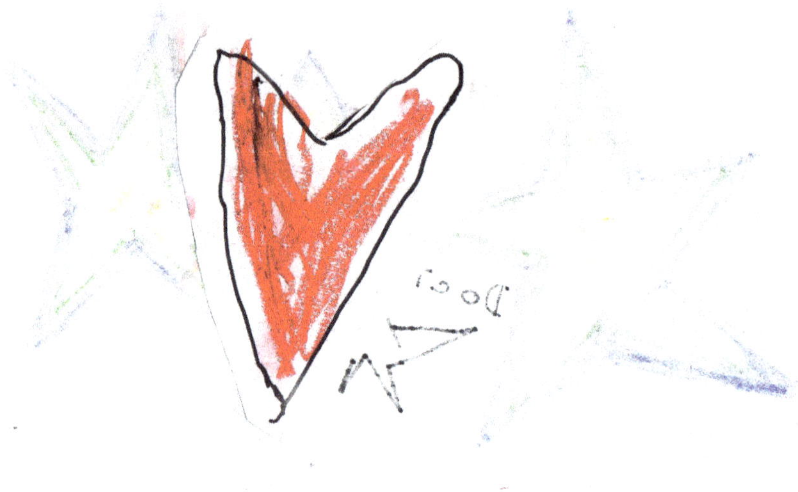

Figure 4.3b Heart

The following vignette occurred amid growing parental conflict about divergent views of Ella's bedtime routine. Mother was concerned that Father would rile Ella with excited, over-stimulating play or at the very least oppose her efforts to help calm Ella. Ella's mother would then try to establish a boundary with Ella's father and with Ella.

As I opened the door to the waiting room, I noticed that Ella seemed to be in a relatively upbeat mood. As her mother rose to depart, they interacted playfully. Ella protested her mother's leave-taking by hugging her leg, but it seemed entirely playful as she cajoled her mother to stay.

MOTHER: I need my leg back. No! No!

ELLA: *(Ella released her grip and darted into the office. Mischievously, she tried to close the door to block me, as if wanting to lock me in the waiting room. Although I had my keys in hand, I worried that this scene could quickly get out of control. This sequence was a first, so I felt completely unprepared. I slipped into the office, while she gently pressed the door against me.)*

ANALYST: *(In a firm and steady voice)* No, No! We don't do that.

ELLA: *(She gently resisted a couple times, but then quickly gave up. She tossed off her shoes and leaped onto the couch.)*
Mamma! Mamma!
(She climbed on to the top of the seat cushions, plunged into the couch head-first, and then began kicking her feet against the back of the couch.)

ANALYST: *(Uncharacteristically, I sat down at my desk chair, momentarily catching my breath to think. I felt de-authorized. I realized that my retreat to my grown-up chair would not serve us well. Hoping to inspire potential engagement, I repositioned myself quickly to one of the small chairs next to the child table, while she remained on the couch several feet away.)*
I think you don't like when I say No. I'm not mad at you when I say no, but . . .

ELLA: *(Talking over me, she spoke quickly and angrily. Her words had decayed so I could not understand them but there was no mistaking that she was upset with me.)*

ANALYST: Oh, I guess you're not ready to hear what I have to say.

ELLA: *(She paused as if trying to listen.)*

ANALYST: I think when I say, "No!" you might think I'm mad at you, or that I don't like you anymore, which is scary.

ELLA: *(She stomped her feet on the couch.)* No! That's not it!

ANALYST: That's not it?

ELLA: *(She jumped off the couch angrily, stomped over to where I was seated, and turned her back to me. She fiercely shook her body from side to side.)*
Grrr! Grrr!

ANALYST: You're really showing me your angry feelings. There is room in here for those parts of you too.

ELLA: Grrr! Grrr!

ANALYST: Grrr! Grrr! Use your words to say what you feel.

ELLA: Stop!

ANALYST: Stop?! You want me to stop talking? Oh.

ELLA: *(A very short while thereafter, she became much calmer.)*

She began to draw a heart. Respecting that she probably wanted quiet, I decided to draw an illustration next to her – a constellation of three stars with her name written above the stars. (The pseudonym "Ella" was inserted to protect confidentiality.) From time to time, she looked over at my picture as I showed interest in her image of a heart. Then she asked if she could color in the stars, added a yellow star between and underneath the large stars, and asked me to write my name above her star.

ANALYST: *(I recognized that she still seemed immersed in the joint construction between us as we approached the end of the session.)*
Ella, I am thinking that we could use this box for projects that we are still working on and that aren't yet complete. We can keep all the supplies you and I are using in here.

ELLA: *(She smiled.)* You read my mind!

ANALYST: Oh! Sometimes you and I come up with great ideas together.

ELLA: *(She continued to cut out the heart she had drawn.)*

ANALYST: I notice you seem much calmer now than you were at the start of the session. Sometimes you're mad at me, and sometimes you're happy.

And today we can see how one feeling turned into another, and now you seem to be very calm.

ELLA: *(She started coloring in the heart, in red.)*

ANALYST: Okay, it is time for us to start cleaning up. *(I began putting away the markers.)*

ELLA: Keep the red pastel out! Now, tape this! *(She helped herself to cotton balls, positioning them behind the heart, which she then placed on the back of the co-constructed illustration. A short while later, the session ended.)*

* * * * *

Many noticeable firsts occurred at this point because language and symbolization could increasingly enable her to use me in an advancing *transference object* role. In the waiting room, Ella hugged her mother's leg as she was accustomed to rough-housing with her father before bedtime. Then she pushed the door frame against me in a show of unprecedented force to press up against my boundaries. Perhaps her mother and I had swapped roles – she related to her mother as if to her father, while Ella challenged me as her internal mother.

Looking back, I thought my illustration unconsciously expressed the family constellation. She had employed me as a symbolic family member. I had placed a small star between two "grown-up" stars, perhaps unknowingly conveying a wish that Ella (as the little star) would feel held by her parental couple (shown by the large stars). I Iined the letters of her name directly along the border of the stars as if I were wishing to provide her with my *internal analytic setting* as a new foundation for her self-development. I wondered: Might Ella have come to feel more secure as the session progressed because we were able to recover from our earlier confrontation, evidenced by her locating herself (by her little star) front and center on the page (or in my mind)? I inferred that she was relying upon me to carry both positive and negative transference dimensions. She chose to add the heart to the underside of our shared drawing, transforming it with the cotton balls into a more fully embodied and enlivened heart. Perhaps she was conveying that our work was gaining momentum, founded by our heart-filled moments together.

These drawings represented the first time that she had allowed us to share artwork, reflecting the deepening of the analysis and the growth in her use of me as both *developmental* and *transference objects*. This vignette captures the way that she was learning to tolerate loving and hating feelings toward the same object, as she moved back and forth between *paranoid-schizoid* and *depressive* forms of relating (Klein, 1935). She was developing a capacity for ambivalence as she gathered more sense of a self that would allow her to recover from distress and disappointment. Spoken communication was now serving as a *container* (Bion, 1962) for her aggression, so we could make psychological sense of her experience to enable further developmental steps. My drawing revealed countertransference attempts to make sense of the transference, recognizing that Ella desperately needed a sense of security that would come from my maintaining the firm boundaries of the analytic setting.

Vignette no. 5

In contrast with the previous vignette, the following session called for me to serve more in role as a *developmental object*, hearkening back to an earlier phase of analysis. By this time, Ella knew well that it was paramount to use words to express her affectionate longings, and yet she still periodically pressed against the boundaries by flying toward me with a hug or wishing to touch my necklace. In this session, I was helpless to resist her impulsive demand to gratify her wish to penetrate my body and mind.

We began by collaborating nicely. As she drew, we sat next to each other at the coffee table on the floor. She allowed me to comment without forbidding me to speak or look at her drawings, also a sign of progress in the analysis as her transference to me as a rejecting object began to soften. Suddenly, she moved over from where she was sitting to rest her face against my leg. Immediately, I pulled my leg away. As I did so, she made brief but forceful contact with me by bumping her body against my leg. She commanded, "Scoot over!" Before I could apprehend what was coming next, she tried to slither under my legs that formed a triangle with the floor. Was she relating to my body as a make-believe bridge that she could crawl under? I tried to reiterate again the importance for us to find words or toys to express her desires and imagined stories rather than using my body as a prop.

ANALYST: Oh, you're wanting to pretend my legs are a bridge. *(I began to stand up.)* No, we need to try to find toys to make a bridge. *(Unbeknownst to me, the palm of her hand was positioned near the heel of my shoe. As I moved forward, she let out a loud cry, followed by a whimper. Shocked, I apologized and expressed concern about her injury. I refrained from speaking again to her misuse of my body so as not to shame her, while locating the responsibility solely within me at this stage.)*

ELLA: *(In a heartbeat, she ran away from me and retreated to the arm of the couch with her back to me. After a brief silence, she reached for the sand tray and brought it back, reclaiming her former seated position next to me. Ever so slowly, she kneaded the sand, looking up at me from time to time with a half-smile.)*

ANALYST: *(As she turned over the sand and self-soothed, I reflected on what I might say. I wondered what she would be able to take in and imagined a complex set of ways that she might have experienced this injury. Had she disowned her aggression by projecting it onto me, only to then experience me as intentionally hurting her? Was she upset at herself for trespassing on my body in ways she knew were not allowed? I spoke slowly, measuring my words and trying to use a gentle, caring tone as I ventured forward in the role as a containing developmental object.)*

Earlier in the session, you and I were playing nicely together, and it seemed as if we were enjoying talking to each other. Then I accidently hurt you. I am very sorry that I hurt you by mistake with the heel of my shoe, but maybe it is not necessary for the good feelings between us to be washed away by that unfortunate event.

ELLA: *(She continued to knead the sand and seemed to be listening intently. We sat together in silence for a few brief moments. Outside my awareness and ever so quickly, she rose and hugged me by gently encircling her hands around my neck from behind.)*

ANALYST: *(As the end of the session neared, she seemed unable to use words to seek reparation for our shared faux pas.)*

Oh, I think maybe you are trying to tell me that you forgive me for what I did and that you like it that we can talk about these things together.

ELLA: *(She resumed her sand play in silence amid a calm atmosphere between us.)*

* * * * *

In this session, Ella was unable to restrain her impulse to express her longing to use my body as a bridge or to hug me, and I felt impotent to protect her from her own urges. As I tried to re-establish the firmness of the boundaries by moving my body away and by invoking the importance of words, I caused her to experience an "injury" that shocked us both. Retreating, she used the sand as a self-soothing device that was a creative and resourceful way to rely upon the setting as a stand-in for me as a *developmental object* that could comfort her even in the face of her hurt and the wedge between us.

I opted against interpreting the transference in that moment as I thought that it would overwhelm her and complicate her anger at me for rejecting her loving feelings, her guilt for her own contribution in producing her hurt, and her ambivalence. It was only near the end of the session that she seemed to gather herself, so I thought she could not make use of a transference interpretation.

At later stages of the analysis, Ella was able to contain her impulse to using my body. For example, she would come running toward me as if about to give me a hug but come to a screeching halt a foot away from me. She became more amenable to directing her affection or aggression into play or to using her words and powerful imagination to communicate her affects.

Vignette no. 6

At earlier phases of the analysis, Ella was unable to verbalize her feelings directly to me as we anticipated separations. We used a calendar to prepare her for such absences and to mark the continuity of our work. On this occasion, in contrast, she was able to create a highly imaginative play narrative that not only conveyed her feelings of longing and sadness but also showed her growth at representing her affection for me through the play rather than through my body.

Ella was about to leave with her family on an atypically long five-day vacation. As I opened the door to the waiting room, she was seated at the child table, quietly

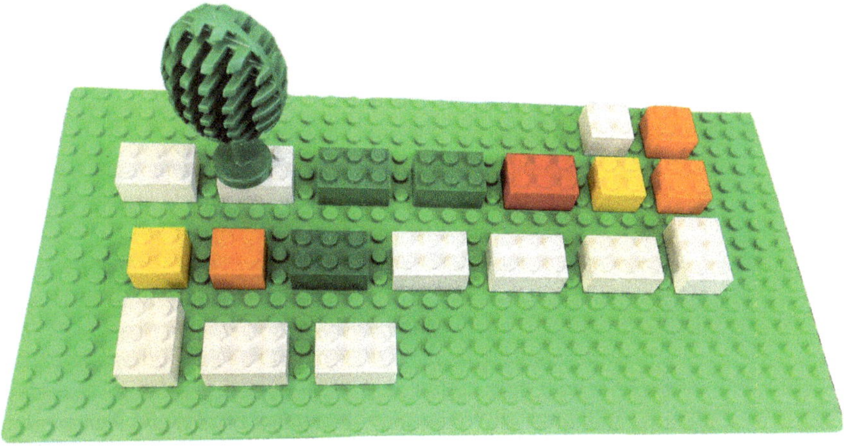

Figure 4.4 Lego project before a separation

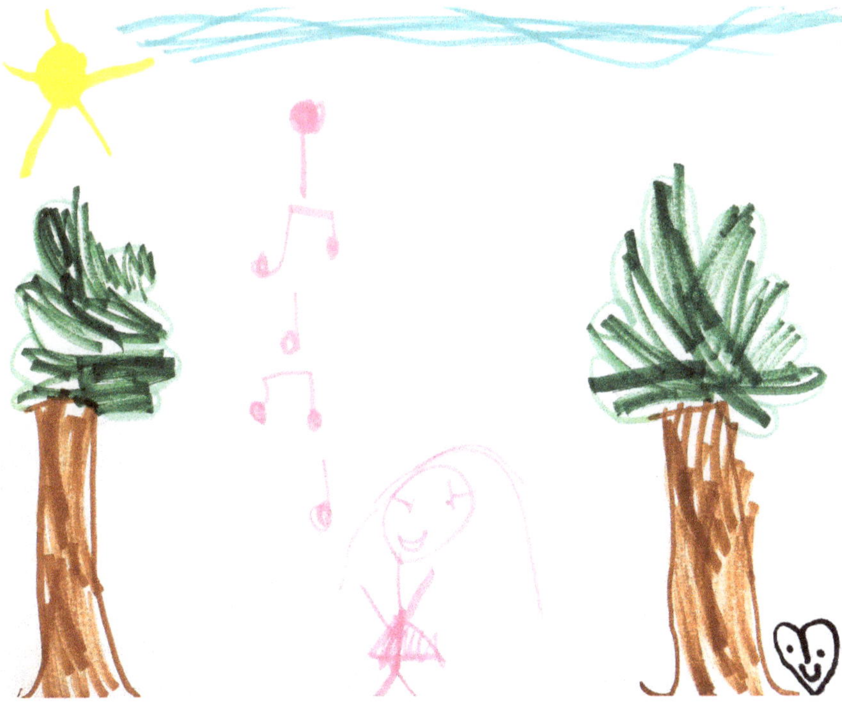

Figure 4.5 Child between two trees

drawing. She remained seated briefly with her head down, neither acknowledging me nor bidding her mother farewell. She finished her drawing quickly, then made her way into the office with her drawing in hand.

ANALYST: *(I closed the door after she entered.)*

ELLA: *(Inside the office, she stood against the child table looking at the toys in a deeply reflective stance. Then she sat down and began tossing the Legos back and forth between her hands without using them to make something at that moment.)*

ANALYST: *(At a recent session, I had assembled the Legos in a sequenced format to represent the sessions progressing through the week as one way to prepare for the upcoming separation. I positioned a Lego tree on a brick to identify the current day and moved it along the bricks to mark the days intervening during the separation.)* This is Tuesday, then we will meet on Wednesday, Thursday, Friday, and then we will be apart from each other for five days.

ELLA: *(She looked at me attentively. Then she showed me her drawing that she had been working on in the waiting room. Ella typically did not wish to discuss her drawings, so I came to regard them much like a dream in a session, where all subsequent commentary could be regarded as associations to the picture or dream.)*

ANALYST: Hmm, you are between two really big trees. Oh! I didn't mean to say that was you. I don't actually know that is you. And there are music notes.

ELLA: *(She nodded her head without uttering any sounds or words.)*

ANALYST: Oh, it is! Yes, you are between two really big trees. And there are music notes too.

ELLA: *(She started to sing.)* La, la, la, la. *(She went to the corner of the office and descended upon a basket that was filled with stuffed animals.)*

ANALYST: It looks like you're giving all the animals a really big hug, but it seems also that you have very strong feelings as you stay there in the corner.

ELLA: *(Ever so slowly, she picked herself up, then caressed and touched the stuffed animals with affection. Slowly fingering the otter's whiskers, she looked over at me. Our gaze met. I was moved by her expression of deep sadness, sensing also that she wanted me to notice her sorrow.)*

ANALYST: As I watched you giving the animals such a big hug, it reminded me of a day when you used to want to give me a hug. Now you're able to do what you couldn't do before, to give the animals a hug and show us your feelings with the toys as I've asked you to.

ELLA: That was what I did when it was a new way *(meaning when we had just started meeting)*, and now I do what is an old way, because now I come here every day *(which was not actually true, as we met Monday through Thursday, for four days each week)*.

ANALYST: Yes, we've come a long way since those early days, when it was a new way, and we still have a long way to go. Now we meet almost every day, and so it can be hard to be apart from one another.

ELLA: *(She returned to the child table while I remained seated a little longer at the couch. She picked up a Lego character.)* This is a police officer.

ANALYST: *(I began to move from the couch to approach her at the child table.)*

ELLA: This is what a police officer does. *(She pointed to the officer's shackles in hand.)* This is what he uses to put a leash on someone, so he doesn't go anywhere.

ANALYST: Oh, so he doesn't go away!

ELLA: Yeah, so he's trapped!

ANALYST: Oh!

ELLA: *(She then motioned aggressively for me to return to the couch.)*

ANALYST: *(I followed her command.)* Oh, you want me to sit here.

ELLA: *(She nodded and sat down on the floor mid-way between the table and the couch, playing with the Legos, while intermittently looking up at me.)*

ANALYST: Oh, now we are further apart *(as she had directed me away from the table to the couch)*, but I can still see you. I can still think about you, and I can wonder about you.

ELLA: *(She proceeded to play quietly, then got up and moved to look out the window.)* Stay there for 155 billion, million days.

ANALYST: 155 billion, million days? Wow! That is a really long time. That would mean that I surely wouldn't move from this couch for the entire time you're gone.

* * * * *

This vignette demonstrates Ella's capacity to use me as a *developmental object*. Feelings about separation could be verbalized rather than merely enacted. When we anticipated separations at earlier phases of the work, her play would typically become quite impoverished. For example, she would count the days on the calendar in a rote way as if she were trying to grasp an unimaginable reality. On this occasion, in contrast, she directed me playfully to return to the couch and to stay for "155 billion, million days." She spoke in a playful tone that lacked the earlier stridency. As we worked through the negative transference to me as a rejecting object and as she seemed to internalize me as a "good-enough" *developmental object*, she anticipated separations with much less anxiety and engaged in more imaginative and collaborative play.

Vignette no. 7

As the analysis progressed, not only was Ella more able to use me more effectively as a *transference object*, but also she was able to receive direct transference interpretations. She built on the work done previously in the displacement of play and as an example of her readiness to receive in-depth transference interpretation. I said: "Oh, I think I get something now. . . . *(She listened very attentively.)* At home, sometimes your mom is in a meeting with someone, and the door to her room is closed. At those times, you're on the other side of the room, all alone, and maybe you feel lonely and hurt that you can't be with her. In here, sometimes you want me to be all alone while you are playing with the toys and the dolls so I know how you feel at home with your mom."

Ella seemed able to take this idea on board, as she immediately engaged her dolls. She disappeared beneath the table to whisper their dialogue between them outside my view. My direct interpretation would not have been received earlier in the treatment, even when she could relate to me primarily as a *transference object*. By this later stage, we had made major forays into many of her conflicts, and the analytic relationship had become strong enough to support deepening of the work.

Conclusion

Ella presented originally with profound developmental delays and a high level of distress. She suffered heightened vulnerability to separation and rejection; she was prone to outbursts with empathic failures; and she was delayed academically due to socio-emotional difficulties. Throughout the treatment, she longed for me to recognize her capacity for growth and resilience, even though her disorganized self leaked out in the form of jumbled words, meltdowns, and enuretic and encopretic episodes. Insecurely and anxiously attached to her parents, Ella contended with a post-traumatic stress syndrome in which she reenacted experiences of rejection toward me in the transference that reflected traumatic family links (Scharff, Losso and Setton, 2017). She expressed conflict about dependency, often stating she was okay when she was hurting or that she could do things all by herself. At times, she aimed to control me by prolonging sessions, or, in reaction formation, she would say, "Oh, good! It's time to go home!" At times, Ella's emotional lability resembled a disorganized style of relating, expressing contradictory feeling, for instance longing for my help while angrily rejecting my offers. Although that feature did not appear frequently, when it did, these discordant wishes were extremely distressing to her.

These challenges were augmented by her speech disturbance, a severe constitutional phonological disorder. For years, Ella felt people could not make sense of her spoken words, despite her efforts to enunciate clearly. She seemed to think people ought to know what she was trying to say, if only people would listen. She was filled with impotence and frustration and often felt unheld and uncontained. Without being able to communicate reliably, she was deprived of this powerful way to regulate strong affects. Ill equipped to interact competently, her sense of self was buffeted by experiencing countless empathic failures. As her communicative efforts were in vain, it was no wonder that she felt pressured to rely only upon herself. Perhaps holding her urine and stool were ways to preserve her internal psychic contents in an external world that often seemed frightening and unresponsive.

Fortunately, Ella was endowed with considerable strengths – her eagerness to relate, her intellect, her symbolic capacities, her determination to communicate strong affects, and her perseverance in the face of misattunement or misunderstanding. All these factors contributed to her resilience in the face of adversity.

I have endeavored to illustrate the highly creative ways in which Ella used me, the office toys, and the analytic setting as *developmental* and *transference objects*. Our work enabled her to advance her development by installing and relating to me as a "good-enough" object (Winnicott, 1965). By redesigning my office into her own open-floor plan, she reconfigured the analytic setting as a potent way to retaliate symbolically against her parents for ways she felt wounded by her sense of their abandonment. In an analogous way, she would repeatedly say to me, "I'm busy now, so I can't talk now!" – turning the transference tables on me. It would be a long time, however, before Ella and I could begin to work directly in the transference in relation to my role as a rejecting object.

My first encounter with Ella offered an initial window into her potential use of me as both *transference* and *developmental objects*. That session represented a harbinger of many salient conflicts and dynamics that subsequently were replayed throughout the analysis. I have provided several vignettes to demonstrate the progression over the course of the analysis from her preferential use of me as a *developmental object* at earlier phases of the analysis to her growing use me as *transference object*s expressed in the displacement of the play or by working with direct transference interpretations. At regressive moments in the analysis, I noticed how she reverted to relying on me as a *developmental object* when she became overexcited or overwhelmed by affects that collapsed her thinking. Over time, she became more capable of utilizing her internal resources to recover from those regressed moments. Gradually, she was able to develop a sturdier psychic organization, working through traumatic experiences by her use of me as both *developmental* and *transference objects*.

Although it was evident that the analytic journey would take still more time, at the stage of these examples, I felt hopeful that she could achieve a significant transformation because of her constitutional strengths, her parents' commitment to the work, and the robustness of the analytic relationship. Ella made these substantive gains largely because of her talented ways of using and creating me, and all possible objects, within the analytic setting. I am grateful to Ella and her family for giving me an intimate sense of her inner world, as she entered my mind en route to finding her own.

References

Baranger, M. (1993). The mind of the analyst: From listening to interpretation. *International Journal Psychoanalysis*, 74: 15–24.

Bernardi, R. (2014). The three-level model (3L-M) for observing patient transformations. In M. Altmann de Litvan (Ed.), *Time for Change: Tracking Transformations in Psychoanalysis – The Three-Level Model*. London: Karnac.

Bion, W. R. (1962). *Learning from Experience*. London: Tavistock.

Chused, J. F. (1988). The transference neurosis in child analysis. *Psychoanalytic Study of the Child*, 43: 51–81.

Fairbairn, W. R. D. (1952). *Psychoanalytic Studies of the Personality*. London: Routledge.
Klein, M. (1935). A contribution to the psychogenesis of manic-depressive states. *International Journal of Psychoanalysis*, 16: 145–174.
Neely, C. (2020, in press). The Developmental Object and Therapeutic Action. *Psychoanalytic Study of the Child.*
Scharff, D. E., Losso, R. and Setton, L. (2017). Pichon Rivière's psychoanalytic contributions: Some comparisons with object relations and modern developments in psychoanalysis. *International Journal of Psychoanalysis*, 98(1): 129–143.
Scharff, D. E. and Scharff, J. S. (1998). *Object Relations Individual Therapy*. Northvale, NJ: Jason Aronson.
Scharff, D. E. and Scharff, J. S. (2011). *The Interpersonal Unconscious*. Lanham, MD: Jason Aronson.
Sehon, C. (2013). The synergy of concurrent couple and child therapies viewed through the lens of link and field theories. *Couple and Family Psychoanalysis*, 3(1): 61–71.
Tähkä, V. (1993). *Mind and Its Treatment*. Madison, CT: International University Press.
Tustin, F. (1980). Autistic objects. *International Review of Psychoanalysis*, 7: 27–39.
Winnicott, D. W. (1965). *The maturational processes and the facilitating environment: Studies in the theory of emotional development*. The Hogarth Press and the Institute of Psycho-Analysis.

5 Analysis interminable

The analyst's self as object for the patient

Nancy L. Bakalar

Over the past four or five years I have developed a particular interest in patients whose treatments seem to have dragged on too long. I am referring to patients who have been in therapy for more than five years, made appreciable gains in their relationships and in work, but then seemed to be stuck. Quinodoz termed these patients "heterogeneous" (Quinodoz, 2001) in that they are capable of secondary process thinking but suffer from unconscious splitting and private periods of misery. Another way to think about them is that they have both pre-Oedipal and Oedipal dynamic issues. In several of my cases, the treatment was at a crossroads: I needed to help each patient move toward termination or to institute a more intensive treatment of psychoanalysis to try to get at the root of the apparent impasse. After many years of practicing, I now offer these patients analysis earlier in their treatment. These are patients whose character structures have at least minimal permeability, so that I have a sense that I *can* be taken in and used as an object, but who seem unable to let themselves fall into close relationships because they are guarded and lack trust. Patients who cannot attach to the therapist or the therapeutic work or whose character structures are so narcissistic and rigid that in the countertransference I feel dehumanized, I have not tried to treat. The patients I describe here are in a category between those who are depressed and/or anxious and those who are unreachable because of severe narcissism or psychosis. These are patients who relate to others socially but suffer internally in that they are not able to love or feel loved, suffer from severe affective distress, and are blocked in their development.

Freud's ideas about interminable cases

Freud wrote about the limitations of psychoanalysis in several major papers. In Lecture XXVIII of the *Introductory Lectures on Psychoanalysis* (Freud, 1917) and in Lecture XXXIV of the *New Introductory Lectures on Psychoanalysis* (Freud, 1933), he seemed to be more optimistic about what might be achieved by psychoanalysis than in his widely read paper *Analysis Terminable and Interminable* (Freud, 1937).

In the later paper, Freud (1937) is more pessimistic about an analytic complete cure. Freud declares, "psycho-analytic therapy – the freeing of someone from his neurotic symptoms, inhibitions and abnormalities of character – is a time-consuming business" (p. 214). He didn't believe all patients could be cured and accepted that failures were inevitable (p. 155). Barriers to cure include what he identified as underlying biological or physiological causes; the constitutional strengths of the (id) instincts; weaknesses of the ego; masochism, meaning the presence of guilt and need or, more specifically, taking pleasure in self-punishment – this latter factor a part of the death instinct.

Hopes for cure vary with whether the psychic conflict arose because of a traumatic experience or was constitutional; the severity of trauma – what Freud termed the quantitative factor; and, finally, the role of the analyst, by which he meant that the analyst "pulls" for the transference. In modern thinking, we pull especially for the negative transference, which is then analyzed and "frees" the patient of his conflicts. In providing the conditions for transference to develop and take hold, the patient's conflicts are de-repressed, that is, come into consciousness, where they can be worked through and, it is hoped, mastered in relation to the analyst.

In this same paper (*Analysis Terminable and Interminable*) Freud (1937) discusses in detail the many limitations of psychoanalysis. Describing the ideal conditions for a successful analysis, he says that the patient's ego has not been "noticeably altered" (damaged) and that the cause of the disturbance was an external factor, that is, traumatic. Presciently, Freud also noted that if an individual sustained trauma at a very young age, when the ego was immature, the patient would be unable to master the trauma; that is, an analysis would likely be unsuccessful or only partially successful. The goal of Freud's analysis was to make the unconscious conscious. That is, repressed conflict is brought into consciousness through the vehicle of the transference, where it can be noted, discussed, worked through, and then repressed again with less conflict. In sum, the goal was to make the unconscious conscious.

More modern analytic theorists have taken up the challenges of treating patients with early, pre-verbal trauma, those who Freud felt were largely untreatable – patients whose trauma occurred at the very beginning of life or before the age of language development, when the child had little or no symbolic thinking. (Only that which can be symbolized can be repressed.) The trauma may have been physical, sexual, psychological, or simply emotional neglect, a chronic or rather sudden cessation of responding to the child emotionally, as in Andre Green's (1972) "Dead Mother Complex," which I will speak to shortly. Patients whose trauma was pre-verbal may present with dread, angst, confusion, rage, or untamed or uncontained affects, now often called Bionian beta bits. In contrast to Freudian analysis, the task in these treatments is to make the conscious unconscious. This is achieved by allowing the patient to express these strong emotional states in sessions, with the analyst naming them, not retaliating, and allowing the patient to "go on being" with the analyst in the wake of affective breakdown and severe attacks on the analyst. The analyst assists the patient in developing alpha function by taking in the patient's raw emotions, or beta bits, inside herself, converting them to alpha bits, symbolized affects, and returning them to the patient in a mentally digested form. This helps structure the patient's mind and brings relief.

Master Speaker Series

The theme of the 2016–2017 Master Speaker Seminar Series at The International Psychotherapy Institute was "The Use of the Self." I presented a paper titled, "The Use of the Self: When the Patient Is Stuck, the Therapist Digs Deeper." In that paper, I emphasized that the therapist needs to take head on the painful transference reactions of the patient which sometimes come as direct attacks. Our task is to absorb them, not fend them off. These transference reactions give us insight into how the patient is feeling, what he is suffering, and by that process itself gives the patient some measure of relief – a sense of being understood. My recommendation in that paper was to view the analytic role as being *active* internally, intrapsychically. I do not mean here to be active in relating to the patient. The theme of our 2017–2018 seminar was "The Use of the Other," and in this chapter, I take up that theme from the perspective of what we as therapists and analysts do to let ourselves be used as *an other*, as an object for traumatized patients, as an instrument in patients' movements toward sturdier character structures, even if not more total cures.

In the 2017–2018 Master Speaker Seminar Series, Charles Ashbach (2017) presented a paper titled, "A Reversible Perspective: Who the Subject? . . . Who the Object?" He said,

> Traumatized patients . . . avoid the pain and [sense of] danger associated with . . . the compromised nature of his/her attachment to the primary objects of infantile experience [which leads] to fears of abandonment . . . and intense feelings of ambivalence that threaten the [patient's] sense of self, security in object-relationships and his/her ability to lead a satisfying and creative life." Ashbach continued, "The patient engages in blockages, confusion and dangers in the process. . . . The term resistance [has been used] to describe such moments in [such a patient's] . . . treatment . . . but we note the dangers involved with [using this term]. . . . The patient 'resists' not because he/she is stubborn or oppositional, not because of . . . [a] . . . Freudian . . . death instinct, but because of the. . . [terror of psychic] danger, of the threat to the [patient's] sanity . . ."

I agree wholeheartedly with Ashbach's comments. The word "resistance" is a packed symbol that needs to be unpacked whenever it arises in the analyst's mind during treatment, in supervisions, or in writing. The idea of "resistance" is a place to *begin* understanding, not foreclose it. In times past, to say a patient was "resisting" often took on a tone of denigration. A patient's resistance has dynamic meaning that needs to be ferreted out! Why is the patient resisting? What is dangerous in this moment? In this process? Between analyst and patient at this moment in the transference?

W. R. D. Fairbairn's theoretical contribution

Fairbairn (1944, 1963) teased out the dynamic mechanisms internal objects influence in the formation of character structure. According to him, being in relationship with a good enough object does not require repression. However, bad object experiences link to parts of the ego, parts of the central self, and, for protection, must be repressed into the unconscious. This maneuver diminishes the sense of self and saps the life-force from the person because, along with the bad object experience that is repressed, the part of the self that is linked to bad objects is also repressed. Patients L and M, described later, intermittently wail about a feeling of not having a "self." These patients often cannot live up to their potential in life or work, their creativity stifled and their ties to others thin and fragile. My countertransference experience with these patients is usually one of my feeling not in a close emotional relationship to them. They have built up a protective shell inside their mind, and so I feel as if I cannot connect with them emotionally, nor does my relating to them seem to touch them affectively.

Here are a few quick sketches of patients who have left me feeling blocked out:

- A patient whose mother was sick from his birth and died when he was a toddler. Basically, he went through life never asking for help. He also played a lot of sports to fill up the emptiness and the loss. I looked for him to attach to me, but he never really did and left treatment prematurely.
- A woman whose mother was cruel and critical, who likely was not able to think symbolically, and whose father was an absent businessman. The patient suffered from hypersexuality and promiscuity and lived a manic lifestyle.
- A man in his early 60s who had recently divorced, lost his job and was sometimes frighteningly suicidal said, "I just want to have fun." Here, the desire to have fun was a desire to fill up the void and cover over the dread of an unconscious sense of being alone. Early in this analysis the man's dreams were also of a psychotic nature in that the elements of the dreams were not linked.
- Patients with a *Dead Mother Complex*. Andre Green (1972) described this psychic situation. It occurs after a child has been in a good (enough) relationship with his mother, and then something catastrophic happens to her. The mother becomes severely depressed and withdraws affectively from the child. Suddenly, the child is related to by an emotionally deadened mother. The lights go out in his world.

Andre Green's Dead Mother Complex

Andre Green's theory (1972) points to a sudden change in the child's caretaker's emotional state. I offer three case examples in which patients suffered with mothers who themselves had Dead Mother Complexes. These mothers could not connect emotionally with their infants and young children. All three mothers seemed (from what I can glean from the patients' treatments) not to have been able to think symbolically – there was insufficient maternal alpha function. To paraphrase Bion (1962), it takes two minds to think one's thoughts. The patients described herein did not have a mother/parent to help them develop their thinking apparatus by mutual projection and introjection and therefore were unable to convert beta experiences to psychological understanding using alpha function. This occurs naturally between infant and mother in good-enough mothering and is the mechanism in therapy and analysis most used in treating patients who suffer in ways described here.

John Steiner's theory of psychic retreats

In his book *Psychic Retreats* John Steiner (1993) took up the study of patients whose intrapsychic organizations spanned characterological types from the normal to the neurotic, borderline, and psychotic. Steiner's experience was that these patients seemed to hide or take refuge in or retreat into an intrapsychic place where they felt protected from anxiety and pain. Quoting Steiner,

> Trauma and deprivation in the patient's history have a profound effect on the creation of pathological organizations, even though it may not be possible to know how much internal and external factors contributed.
>
> (p. 8)

These mechanisms are present to a greater or lesser extent depending on the health of the individual. In severe forms of pathological organizations, the patient's mind is in shambles. While healthier patients intermittently feel overwhelmed with anxiety and an inability to think, they are only transiently unable to shake their minds free of collapse. At the more ill end of the spectrum, those patients who have less mental scaffolding to draw upon, individuals experience the internal attack of repressed bad objects as coming from the outside. It is the splitting and repression of self and object; under stress, the patient feels obliterated or annihilated. Quoting Steiner,

> These [psychic] organizations are conceptualized as both a grouping of defenses and as a highly structured, close-knit system of object-relationships.
>
> (p. xi)

Steiner continues,

> Sometimes the retreat is experienced as a cruel place . . . but more often the retreat is idealized and represented as a pleasant and even ideal haven.
>
> (p. 2)

This defensive system offers the patient protection from the fear of annihilation – and therefore there is resistance to giving it up, even though patients suffer immensely.

> It is as if the patient has become accustomed and even addicted to the . . . [psychic] retreat and gains . . . perverse gratification from it.
>
> (p. 12)

This harkens back to Freud's death instinct and to the ideas he put forward in *Analysis Terminable and Interminable* (Freud, 1937). Freud would have viewed this pathological defensive mechanism as "constitutional" rather than due to external trauma; as nature, not nurture.

Case of L

I met L about 15 years ago when she sought me out to manage medications for her anxiety and depression. L worked and was reliable in her job. After several years of beginning treatment, she married and remains so. So, she functioned well enough in the world. Most of her leisure was spent reading books or watching TV or movies. She never talked about what she was reading or what she saw on TV. I came to realize that this was a symptom of her psychic retreat to literally mind-numbing activities. Intermittently she had horrible, abusive arguments with her partner.

L's developmental history was traumatic. Both her parents grew up with trauma in their own families of origin. Her parents were of the hippie generation and thought it was fine to "let it all hang out!," which they did with their children. When L was a toddler and her mother returned to college, L was left with her father as caretaker. He took her into the shower and exposed her to pornographic materials. Her mother neither intervened nor set limits. Then and now L says that she liked this sexualized relationship with her father. She learned to masturbate at age four or five. Only recently in her analysis were new details revealed: at age seven she remembered being on the parental bed with her father, mother, and brother. They were all looking at pornographic magazines. She became aroused and was both excited and horrified by this in the presence of her parents. She believed her parents knew she was aroused. As her treatment unfolded, it became apparent that her mother had minimal alpha function, minimal ability to think symbolically, and so there was no way for L to think about her overstimulated and confused feelings and bodily sensations.

Treatment

In the early years of treatment, L suffered severely without being able to verbalize her proto-feelings. I also could not put words to them, because she had no words for them. I just saw the suffering and must admit that, sitting in the therapist's seat, I was none too eager to get close affectively. She often bent over from the waist, holding her head, shaking it from side to side, and said with profound angst, "Bees are buzzing in my head." She could not bear for me to speak, move, take a sip of tea, even breathe. She often held up her hand like a traffic cop to stop me from speaking. All my movements reminded her that I was alive, a person. She wanted, perhaps needed, me to be a statue, dead, non-living. This would be in keeping with her murderous desire to kill me as representing the bad object and resonated with all the bad objects she had deadened inside her.

As Ferro (2003) described in his paper on his patient Marcella, the first four or five years with L were spent building – as much as possible – some psychological foundation to help her begin to think; a psychic structure that could tolerate affects, my being not only alive but also a separate individual with my own needs and desires. I offered myself as an object for her transference as a dependable figure with a reliable frame. I bore her attacks. I named feelings for her. For years, she sobbingly railed at me for doing so: "I hate having feelings!" This was consistent with Steiner's (1993) conceptualization of the psychic retreat – a walled-off place where feelings can be numbed or evacuated into the unconscious and from which the patient does want to be pried loose. L did not want to suffer her feelings.

L made appreciable progress during the first five years of twice-weekly therapy, as was evidenced by less anxiety and more empathy with people at work. However, she still suffered severely and continued to escape into mindless activities. I offered, and she accepted, psychoanalysis about seven years ago. About four years ago, she made a very personal attack on me. I was stunned but stayed silent. By the next day she apologized profusely. She was able to sense me as another person who could be hurt. At that moment she was oscillating between the paranoid-schizoid and depressive positions. She truly understood she had hurt me and made amends to repair. She was terrified that I would drop her as a patient. After that, she never made a direct, personal attack on me again.

The next dynamic issue that emerged was her despair and rage that I was not her mother. By then, an experienced patient, she sensed a great difference between how I listened and responded to her and how her mother, with whom she spoke often, did so. She understood the reality that she was not born to me, but she shook her fist at the universe in rage and despair. Another dynamic during this period was that any comment or interpretation that I offered linked up in the transference to her critical, demanding father – and so, for a long time, I was not allowed to make interpretations. That transference reaction still is present intermittently, although she catches herself and realizes her reaction is in response to the old experiences with her father and not to me. Then she is able to pull back the projection and somewhat grudgingly invites the interpretation.

Finally, an erotized dynamic emerged. It started some years before in that L told me she got aroused in the presence of her male boss and then with her female friends and her minister. Then she said she was aroused almost all the time in the presence of anyone. The arousal entered the consulting room. This was extremely painful for both of us. She wanted to touch me sexually. She wondered what my body looked like. She believed I was aroused in her presence – a projection. Later she talked about wanting to be in my womb, as she termed it, and wanting "to relate to me from [her] vagina." (As an aside, the confusion about names of the genital body parts and anatomy, I believe, is a symptom of the hysteric mind – a mind which cannot think.)

Revealing these wishes left her with considerable distress. By this time, I was seeing her by video-teleconferencing because I had moved to another state. This seemed to make bearing the erotized transference easier for both of us. Initially in the countertransference, I felt disgusted and was repelled – not able fully to offer myself as an object for her use. Taking her in felt too sexual. Then, in my reverie, I could picture her being on the changing table as a baby and her dad or mother looking primarily at her genitals and not into her eyes and cooing at her. I said to her, "I think you want others to look at your face, to look into your eyes and to see *you,* not be seen in a sexual way." She sighed, "Yes!" and then said, "And I want to relate to you from my heart and my mind, too, not from my genitals." Internally I sighed with relief because it seemed some understanding had come through these links.

We worked on these issues for a couple of years, but L seemed not to be able to make appreciable use of them; there was no evidence of significant transformation, even though her functioning in the external world was improving. She got a higher-paying job; she felt stronger inside; she was getting along with her family members better, showing more empathy toward her children. She had allowed her friends and family to come alive and no longer needed to turn them into statues.

L had come to my home state once before to see me in person, but on that first occasion I saw her for one session two days in a row. I then suggested she come out for a weekend so we could work intensely together for seven hours per day, from 10 a.m. to 6 p.m., with an hour break for lunch. She was surprised, maybe slightly shocked: "You would do this for me?! You would give up your Sunday for me?!" "Yes," I replied.

This treatment suggestion was modeled after the technique Bollas described in his book *Catch Them before They Fall* (2013), a technique used for patients who were on the brink of breakdown and psychic collapse. Bollas stated that he would cancel patients to make himself available for up to three days. This intensive treatment had been successful in averting a collapse and (as I understood it) strengthened the patient's psychic structure.

L agreed to the offer. We settled on meeting seven hours on a Sunday and three hours on Monday morning. Once she was there, I began to feel vulnerable and scared, feelings that I had not experienced when I had arranged this. Retrospectively, I now understand that these feelings were both a countertransference reaction and a realistic one. In the countertransference, I was feeling what she felt with me and what in her childhood she had felt in the presence of her father. From a reality perspective, I was seeing a woman with an erotized transference on a Sunday, all day, in an otherwise almost empty office building, and my analytic sofa was actually an upholstered twin bed! What allowed me to proceed was that I had worked with her for more than a decade; there was a good alliance; and she accepted boundaries although they made her angry – so I felt comfortable enough to proceed.

Thoughts and plan for my approach to the extended session

I held in mind that L had been excessively sexually and affectively stimulated as a very young child, that the sexual stimulation had overwhelmed her, and, at that young age and because neither parent seemed to have symbolic thinking, she had had no way to think about the confusing physical and psychical sensations. Because I saw her trauma as primarily pre-verbal, I had offered her the extended time, the space of my office, and the space of my mind to use as she needed. I waited and hoped it would be helpful.

Summary of the extended day

L showed up on time Sunday morning well prepared. She had brought all she thought she might need, including bottled water and lunch. She dressed in a forest green sweater set, a long black skirt, and black boots, and she carried a maroon purse. This outfit mimicked a sweater set that I wear often with black pants, and my everyday carry-all bag is the same maroon. When a patient and I show up in the same colors, especially several days in a row, I take it as a sign that we are in good conscious and unconscious resonance in the therapeutic endeavor.

L chose to sit on the regular sofa in the main treatment room, facing me. I asked her if she minded if I took notes. She replied, "No, because then I know you are really listening to me!" This was a momentous day for me, venturing into a treatment modality that I had been interested in for a long time without an opportunity to try it out. Later in the day, I realized that, by taking notes hour by hour, I would have documentation in case there were any accusations of a sexual nature that might arise in L's fantasy but might seem real to her.

L chose to use the regular sofa in various ways. Sometimes she sat up facing me; sometimes she lay down as in analysis; and sometimes she lounged with her legs on the sofa but facing me. It felt important to give her freedom of movement without comment. I just noted the shifts to myself.

L's dream

She started with a dream: "I was in a hotel room. There was noise in the hall. There was food on the floor. I didn't know how it got there. I thought it was a ghost, but that didn't make sense. It was the end of the world. I didn't know why. I was holding my young child's hand. . . . Then there was a medicine bottle with pieces of pills in it. The little girl opened it. She swirled some pieces and pill dust with her finger and put them in her mouth. I told her, 'No!' I swept my finger through her mouth. I'm not sure I got all the pieces out. But I was with a young, blond doctor (it was you!) who could help me. I then realized the child was not my daughter. The face was long and gaunt. It was my face as a young girl, but gaunt, like the painting 'The Scream.' *(She sits up and looks away.)* I'm here. I don't feel I'm here. All these damn layers of defense I need in order to accept your presence."

N: My presence is different?

L: It's awful. What I most want is what I'm most frightened of. It causes me great pain. *(She looks at me.)* I have no doubt you're in me . . . *(she holds her chest)* the internal Nancy has great difficulty soothing the core of the core. *(A few minutes later, crying and leaning away:)*

L: Your presence scares the crap out of me. *(She actually suffers from what she terms "fecal leakage.")* I can't talk to you like a regular person. I noticed you were slightly limping. I can't ask you about it, and if I did, I'd be afraid of the answer.

N: You can ask.

L: How's your knee?

N: It is still sore.

L: I'm afraid to ask questions. I might be rejected.

N: I know.

L: My goal was to lie on your analytical couch. . . . I'd like to just rest on your couch if that's okay. I don't see how I'm going to be able to do that without traumatizing myself. . . . It's a couch, just a couch. *(She stands up and looks at the analytic sofa in the other room.)* I don't trust you.

N: I know.

L: *(Crying.)* It's not personal.

N: I know.

L: I don't trust you after so many years. I don't trust my mom. My dad is dead. I don't trust myself.

(A bit later:)

L: I'm having the arousal feeling and the wrist symptoms *(A feeling of cutting her wrists, which she has never done)* . . . no matter what I am talking about.

N: I want to hear about it. *(Here I am opening myself up to be the object for her projections even though in the past I shrank from it.)*

L: When I tell you about my bodily sensations, it interrupts relating to you – it's about the body instead of about the relationship. *(Sitting up facing me)* . . . It's about being in your space . . . that helps me . . . this is a patient's dream . . . to have you all day. . . . *(The language is infantile and sexual.)*

Highlights of the session

Now I will condense a considerable amount of material that was explicitly sexual, material that I had to open myself up to, again, to serve as the object for her fantasies and projections, so that the important dynamic work had a platform for discussion and thinking.

Sitting up, L repeated her childhood sexual experiences of being exposed to pornography with her parents and her desire to touch her parents' genitals and the arousal and guilt that desire caused. She spoke of how she would sneak into their bedroom to look at the pornography and then steal back to her room behind the bed to masturbate. She felt betrayed and angry that her mother did not protect her from her father. She linked these old experiences to the analytic sofa, how terrified she was to use it and how disappointed she was with herself that she could not.

N: You're afraid.

(She notifies me that she is aroused and immediately asks, "When's lunch?" I tell her whenever she chooses. She says she wants to run away.)

Then:

L: I want to have a relationship with you. . . . Oh! Just then, I got aroused.

N: You equated the relationship with me to a sexual relationship.

L: Yes! But the original thought was pure! It just got sexualized in my mind. . . . Now the two are intertwined – the pure desire for a relationship with the sexualized relationship. . . . *(thinking for a moment)* . . . That was the first time I've been able to separate it. *(She continues around the betrayal of her parents encouraging her to have these sexual experiences because they were "natural.")*

L: And when I showed anxiety, I was chided and mocked!
(A few minutes later).
I cannot go to the analytic couch because it will symbolize that I want to have sex with you. *(She is now lying down on a regular sofa in the therapy room.)* I have a fantasy and desire that you [would] come over and perform oral sex. . . . *(I brace myself; this is difficult for me.)* Apologetically: I'm aware this is part of the work. . . . I feel this is futile. . . . I feel hopeless and helpless. . . . It's a part of me. . . . It's my psychology, in my body, in my life. . . . *(She has been going on for a few minutes, and I decide it is important for me to open up more space for thinking about this . . . although it feels risky.)*

N: What would it be like for me to perform oral sex?

L: Frightening and fantastic! *(Then:)* Did you have to ask that?! Was that important?

N: Yes.

L: Why?! You made a mistake. . . . Now my mind is even more . . . *(pause)* maybe it wasn't a mistake. *(Crying)* . . . I desire you. I want to take you in. . . . *(She sits up.)* No! my dad lost his license because he asked a client to masturbate in his office. . . .

N: *(I interrupt)* . . . I'm not asking you to masturbate . . . I'm asking what it would mean to you.

L: That's how you would love me and I would enjoy it. . . . Because it was sexually exciting. *(Pause.)* Now I am angry at you!

N: *(I feel in danger now.)* It feels very dangerous!

L: I feel taken advantage of. . . .

N: I'm not interested in you sexually. I'm here to help you with these things that keep you anxious and unhappy.

L: I don't believe you! How are you not sexually aroused?! I'm so angry with you!

N: We are not the same person. I don't feel what you feel. *(She goes back to my question of what it would mean to her.)*

. . .

L: *(She is sitting up.)* It would be what I wanted all along . . . a re-enactment with dad and mom. This feels extremely dangerous. It would be the only way I could know they cared about me. . . . It would be the only way I could take them in . . . the only way I could take *you* in . . . the only way! *(She pauses.)* Very lonely, you know. . . . The only way I can let you in is in a sexual way. . . . So I have to block you out. . . . Interesting, it's oral sex . . . oral suckling my genitals. . . . The only way of affection, nourishment, communication . . . like suckling at the breast. . . . Everything I hold most dear is locked up, hidden – too dangerous to give since it is sexual – so it is just locked away . . . [the sexual interaction] is how I could receive what a mother should give her daughter *(affection)*. . . . It's not the healthy, productive way. . . . What I needed was cooing, talking and sharing laughs. . . . Yeah! I was pretty cheated. . . . I have a fantasy of having oral sex on you . . . that would be my way to suckle you. *(Here we see that infantile need/desire/form of attachment gets/got sexualized.)* Does that answer your question?

N: You've done a lot of work in the last 15 minutes.
L: I'm really angry at you . . . *(pause)* . . . I'm making snarky remarks in my head.
N: You're mocking the process?
L: Yes! *(She lies back down, covers her eyes, and rests.)*

Request to take a nap

(After working through the sexual material:)

L: I feel so embarrassed – what I said. I feel like I have ruined our relationship.
N: This is the purpose of our work together.
L: I know . . . I feel so tired. I want to talk . . . I want to sleep . . . I want to run.
N: You can set the pace.
L: I want to sleep. Can I sleep on the sofa?

She lay on the regular sofa and then asked for a blanket. I had an afghan, which I handed to her, ensuring that I did not cover her with it. That would have been too intimate. I asked if she would like me to sit quietly in my usual chair while she slept or if she would like me to work quietly at my desk. She preferred the latter, for which I was grateful. She slept lightly for most of an hour, deeply for a brief interval. I felt like a mother watching over her infant or toddler napping, keeping an ear out for noises she made, what they might mean. Was she sleeping restfully? From my position ten feet away she heard the gentle tapping of the keyboard, which I thought might be soothing to her.

In the remainder of the session, pre-verbal/pre-Oedipal and verbal/Oedipal and post-Oedipal dynamics were present simultaneously. During this extended session, moment to moment, I was most aware of staying focused on keeping the literal space and the space in my mind open for her infantile dynamics. In reviewing my notes, I can see that overtly I was dealing with the predominant sexual Oedipal material and with some interpersonal boundary confusions. However, the pre-Oedipal issues were embedded in the behaviors and processes between us.

Keeping in mind, managing, and responding to L's pre-Oedipal dynamics

How did I attend to her pre-Oedipal dynamics? I gave her considerable freedom in time and space. The only things we had agreed upon ahead of time were that we would meet for seven hours and take an hour lunch break. She chose when we took breaks and for how long and when to take a break for lunch. I allowed her to move about the three rooms (the waiting room, the regular treatment room, and the analytic room) as she chose. She was free to sit up and face me, lie down in analytic style, or lounge. She was free to walk around. At one point, she stood in the doorway between the treatment room and the analytic room and said, "I just can't go in there." I immediately understood that the analytic room stood for her parents' bedroom. I said, "That's fine."

The main treatment room is long and rectangular. My desk and bookcases are at the far end. At one point she got up and wandered to that end of the room and began staring at my diplomas. When she seemed to be reading them too closely, I asked her not to. Why? Because of the multiple names I have on various diplomas, which I thought would stimulate questions about me and would contaminate her treatment. She accepted the limitation fairly easily.

The rooms of my office represented the mother's body. Allowing her the freedom in time and space to walk around in it was as if she were exploring the mother's/the analyst's body. We allow children in play therapy to move about the room, to use the space to work on their dynamic issues. So, too, when we are in the throes of working on pre-Oedipal issues with adults, they need full access and use of space and time within the boundaries of the session. These movements need to be understood but usually not interpreted. To deny movement would re-create the trauma the young child experiences when prohibited from doing something she needs to do to explore a psychological issue. For the analyst to think that the patient is resisting by getting up would be an error in understanding and technique.

Managing and responding to L's Oedipal dynamics

From her neurotic part, L talked about her anxiety about lying on the analytic sofa, how it reminded her of her parents' bed where she was overstimulated, of their betrayal and her hatred of them for that, and of me in the transference because I even have an analytic "bed" to offer her. She talked about her desire to touch her parents' genitals and her interest in mine. She suffered arousal much of the session. She spoke of her wish to have sexual experiences with me. Now, at this stage in my career and experience, I was able to open myself up to the analytic endeavor, to offer myself as an object to better understand what her sexual desires for me (and everyone else!) meant. I was both surprised and pleased to see that her desire for oral sex linked so directly to the infantile wish to be held, nourished, and loved. In several analytic cases I have found links between a disturbance in the infant/toddler relationship with the parents, poorly developed or absent alpha function, inappropriate sexualization of relationships, and sexual perversions.

Follow-up sessions

L had to return to the east coast Sunday night because of a storm. In Monday's session by video link, she was exhausted, embarrassed about all that she had said, and angry at me for it. She was distraught. Tuesday's session was the most integrated, thoughtfully linking session she had ever had. It was as if she were functioning as her own analyst:

L: I am ready to work. The work is how I feel sexual toward you and want a sexual relationship with you . . . and how the fantasy interferes with my getting help from you. . . . I now have a better sense of this fantasy. . . . I know the more I talk about it the more you can help me. . . . This fantasy has become so big . . . but it is just a fantasy . . . so, I try to turn off my feelings, but they come out any way . . . I didn't get the nourishment at the breast – I got it at the crotch . . . my dad's penis at eye level in the shower when I was four . . . at the mouth level. . . . It feels like that was all that was offered . . . my wires got crossed.

N: Your infantile longings got sexualized as you became older . . . at age four, five, six. . . .

L's current work

As I write, two and one-half months have passed since L's day-long session. L still struggles, but, overall, I see her thinking as much more integrated and symbolic. When I met her about 15 years ago, she functioned in the world but had psychotic thinking. She has developed the capacity to name her feelings, although she still resents having to bear them. She no longer walls others off in her unconscious or kills them off by making them "statues." She is insightful and self-analyzes well. She has internalized a faint to moderate sense of me as an object that she can call upon to soothe herself. She has had set-backs in being able to give a narrative of her feeling states. She is struggling with mourning. I hope that once she can mourn more reliably, her internal objects will be more available to her. As Hanna Segal said in *Dream, Phantasy and Art* (1991, p. 40), "A symbol is like a precipitate of the mourning for the object."

Case of M

M is a 45-year-old plain-dressing woman, the oldest of eight children and daughter of a senior church leader. Her father was blustery, critical, demanding, and himself fraught with anxiety. Her mother was a largely non-thinking woman who could not keep up with the workload of the large family and taking care of the family business while the father spent most of his time tending to church matters. Religious teachings include not spoiling children, not allowing them to cry, paying little attention to them, and employing corporeal punishment. More serious issues, such as sexual abuse, are "swept under the rug." The family was poor. Food was scant and of poor quality. There were insufficient clothes.

M sought treatment about 12 years ago. She was bedridden with anxiety and depression and suffered panic attacks. She continued with me by telephone and then by video-teleconference when I moved to another state. I treated her in therapy for several years and then offered and she accepted analysis about six years ago by video technology.

In the analysis, we pieced together an understanding that with her father's loud, frequent, thunderous outbursts and because of her mother's inability to physically and emotionally contain her and the general inattention of being left in the crib to cry much of the time, she was left in a state of fright much too often. She developed an obsessional style, one of "doing" to solve emotional problems, unable to think symbolically. Through the analysis she had a difficult time feeling close to me or, despite my many years of treating her, feeling that I cared about her. She suffered from Steiner's (1993) "gang" of repressed bad objects.

She did well in analysis. After five years or so, she was able to function as a thoughtful mother and to do her work more easily, was less obsessional, and took on important social projects in the community. But recently she suffered a return of severe anxiety and fears of rejection, set off by two family issues: one involved her father, who she felt would put an end to her community project, and the other related to her son, whom she feared would get a rejection letter from a young woman he wanted to date and with whom she overidentified around feelings of rejection.

Her recent anxiety was not as severe as that she experienced five years before but was quite disturbing. Earlier in the analysis, I was identified with the critical, demanding father. Now I was identified with the unhelpful mother who couldn't understand and was not capable of helping her. M feared she would be "too much for [me]" and that I would never be enough for her.

She asked for double and extra sessions. So, for a while I saw her up to ten hours weekly. As with L, this increased intensity of sessions was in line with tending to her infantile needs, a kind of "feeding on demand." As with L, I allowed M the freedom to sit up, lie down, and move around the room. Patients who are working in the pre-Oedipal dynamics desire and need to see the analyst's face. They are looking for the mirroring and to be understood. Also, as with L, I kept the time boundaries.

In one of these sessions, M reported that she had difficulty sleeping, instead tossing and turning. Then she said, "In the middle of the night, I thought of you and held you close to me and that gave me some relief." So, here we see evidence of internalizing the good object experience with me as analyst, as a source of comfort, even though the description of it has a concrete quality.

Soon after this, M needed to get up. She placed her laptop on the coffee table, pointing it down the room, and then I saw her pace agitatedly back and forth for a few minutes and look out the window briefly. She may have been speaking or not. I don't remember. The most important part was to see her. When she stopped, I said to her, "M, it looks like you were feeling like an out-of-sorts, unhappy toddler needing to be picked up and soothed." She agreed. After a few minutes she wanted to lie down. She put the laptop on the floor and lay in front of it, on her stomach, her head toward me. Her arms were down by her sides. Then, surprisingly, she put her forehead on the carpet, appearing to balance her head in that position. I was startled in that she didn't even use her forearms to rest her head on.

N: *(In the countertransference I have the fantasy of a downed soldier playing "possum," pretending to be dead so as not to be shot at or further injured.)* M, you look like a dead soldier on the battlefield.

M: *(She gets up, looks at the camera, and, crying, says:)* That is the lowest I can go! That's what I felt like growing up – lying flat, waiting to be picked up. I felt totally annihilated.

N: Dead.

M: *(She is sobbing now. She has never vocally cried before in the many years that I have known her.)*

N: You needed me to see all that to better understand what you experienced and suffered.

M: Yes. *(Then there is a calmness in her voice, and her facial expression seems almost totally relaxed. Then she surprises me and says:)* Good-bye! *(as if addressing her father. Then, smiling:)* I've got a life to live! *(and she waves her arm away as if dismissing and banishing her father in a tone of "Enough with you!")*

She struggled over the next week, wrestling with her anxiety and obsessions, worried that she would never get well, that she would be burdened by her anxiety for the rest of her life. Then, a week later, on a Thursday, she asked me for extra time on Friday and over the weekend. I found an hour for her on Friday. She said, "What about Saturday?" I told her that I couldn't. She seemed slightly surprised, anxious, but accepted it. Why did I deny her the extra time on Saturday? Because I couldn't be a bottomless pit for her, because I was tired, because I had many things to get done over the weekend, and because I wanted to set a limit and see what she would do with it. The timing of this seems to have been good. She did a lot of thinking, linking, and solidifying her insights. She reassured herself that she had all that she needed in the way of real and emotional supplies, that she had been strong and productive these past five years, and that she didn't need to be a slave to her internalized, demanding father and absent, dead mother (Green, 1972). Wednesday, she was able to link her infantile, toddler, young child, and adolescent family experiences with her symptoms in relation to her parents and to me in the transference. That day, I was once again a good-enough analyst.

Although I am not completely sure, I believe she is in the last stages of her analysis and that this last regression, though fairly short-lived, was a recapitulation of her life struggles and an opportunity to finally anchor her insights, transformations, and success. I believe what was powerful here is that M, like L, had to *show* me her pain – not tell me about it. I had offered the freedom and space to do so – in the room and in my mind. And through that process she could experience me as someone who cared about her, as a good analyst, as a good object, as a good parent. Her bad object experiences have been detoxified, not completely but significantly. And because parts of Fairbairn's Central Self are linked to bad object experiences and repressed into the anti-libidinal ego, detoxifying and freeing the bad object also releases the lost parts of the self, a self that she can now sense and appreciate and for which she was grateful.

Case of P

P is a 77-year-old married man who came for treatment about four years ago, suffering with marked anxiety, depression, low motivation for life, low energy, and fear of death. His anxieties related to violent fantasies of attacking his wife or other women with knives or guns. He suffered poor self-esteem, and consequently, in relation to me, even during the evaluation sessions, he wanted to demonstrate that he was smarter than me.

Developmental history

P was the fourth of five children. He has a sister about six years older and a brother who is two years younger. A sister and a brother, born in the years between his older sister and himself, are deceased. His parents divorced when he was four or five, establishing him as an Oedipal victor. His natural father was alcoholic and emotionally abusive and shaming. P described his mother as full of life, vivacious, hard-working, and admiring of accomplished men. She worked to support herself and the children after the divorce. He admired and loved his mother, really believing she "knew everything." In fact, she could not tolerate his moodiness and mocked his tears, chiding him, "You look ugly when you cry!"

His mother worked when he was a child, and he was left alone in the care of his older sister. He described being sad and forlorn as a boy. He didn't leave the house or play when his mother was away. He wanted to be there as soon as she returned. When his mother did come home, tired and distressed, she secluded herself in her bedroom resting, pushing him away.

His mother dated during his latency, and he and his sibs were left with an aunt for weekends and sometimes weeks at a time, which he resented. His rage toward his mother was exemplified by his holding a young female cat hostage for three days without food or water, then repeatedly making the cat swim across a stream and finally, with his neighborhood friend, stabbing her to death. There was also sexual stimulation in the home. His mother took him into bed with her when he was sick, walked through the house with just her underwear on, and was not private about her monthly periods. Poignantly, he found a pair of her "falsies" in the trash can and carried them in his pockets for a while. He was precociously sexual with neighborhood girls from the age of ten.

Through our work together, it became apparent that his mother did not possess significant alpha function. She taught her children how to live by mottos! A penny saved is a penny earned! Waste not, want not! His mother remarried when he was 13, and so he was displaced permanently by his stepfather during his adolescent Oedipal phase.

When he was 18, he married and moved to a neighboring state to go to college. He then had an emotional breakdown and briefly had to be hospitalized. He missed his hometown and his mother and had developed violent fantasies of stabbing his wife or other young women in the community. Shortly thereafter, he moved back to his home state, finished college, and became a professional. He stayed married but was emotionally abusive toward his wife. He was somewhat of an underachiever in his professional life because he always felt inferior to "alpha" males, the real go-getters.

He had extended psychotherapy treatment with someone who was not dynamically skilled. He developed a crush on her, really became possessed by her. She stimulated his fantasies, and there were mild indiscretions, such as mutual gift-giving and kissing on the cheek. She also shared her personal history of recent divorce and encouraged his fantasies, and so, once again, he was an Oedipal victor!

As soon as treatment started with me, he had violent and sexual fantasies about me. The violent fantasies subsided almost completely after we worked on their early life origins. However, he developed a crush on me and was quite angry that I held the treatment boundaries and would not budge on what he called my "program." I offered and he accepted analysis about one year in to treatment.

For this patient, this sexual fantasy life continued into and lasted throughout his adulthood, to fill the void created primarily by the "dead mother" emotional experience; by his mother's real absences and brush-offs; and, originally, by his father's meanness and then later by his father's real absence.

A session from a year ago

P: I think about you all the time. This morning I was in the shower and . . . *(I immediately get an icky feeling – it feels like something sexual.)* I was washing under my arms, and I thought, "I wonder if Nancy washes under her arms?"

N: *(My first thought is, 'Of course, I do!' Then I think, why armpits? Where is this going? I feel uncomfortable. Then I think, armpits are near the breasts and think of the absent breast, the absent mother, her absent attention . . . the bad breast that needs to be washed.)*

P: I think about you no matter what I am doing. . . . If I am eating breakfast, I wonder, "Is Nancy eating her breakfast? Does she eat cold cereal?" If I am reading, I think of you sitting and reading. I picture you with your husband, but sometimes I picture I am your husband and you are with me . . . that you are mine. . . .

N: *(I am still feeling a little creeped out. I feel taken over inside with what he is saying, just as he describes I have taken over his mind. However, that he "sees" me and thinks about me in so many different places gives me a clue.)* I think you think about me in all these places as a way to keep me close to you. It is as if you want the thought of me to fill up the empty space, the void that creates so much longing and the void that has left you feeling alone, anxious and lonely. . . .

P: Yes! That is exactly right, Nancy. *(And with this both arms arch out to his sides and he brings his arms together and clenches his fists.)* I just want to grab you and take you inside me and hold on to you. *(This is an enactment of his need and desire, as we saw L's and M's enactments in their sessions.)*

N: Yes! I see that. It is to fill the empty, longing space. . . .

P: I think about you all the time . . . I think of your voice, how much I like it. I think of how you look. . . .

N: You like my voice because it is soothing to you. . . .

P: Yes, that's right. and I like that you're smart because I want to be seen as smart, too. *(This comment speaks to his desire to internalize the analyst/mother and be like her.)*

Offering myself as an object for repair ten months later

The patient had been talking about the anxiety and a void he had experienced his whole life and had been reminiscing about his most recent therapist, a woman with whom he had been infatuated.

P: Today when I was getting ready to come here, I took a shower and I was putting on my underwear, "Body Armor," and I was thinking it would really be cool if Nancy could see me. . . .

N: What would be so cool about it? *(Here I invite the details of the erotized transference.)*

P: Well, Body Armor is really cool . . . first of all they are spandex and they have a pouch! I would like you to see how I fill out the pouch. . . . *(He is embarrassed as he describes this.)*

N: *(In my mind I "run" from the image. He has made me feel like a voyeur. I then visualize little kids 2½ to 3½ years old running through the house naked, proud of their bodies, wanting their parents, especially the parent of the opposite sex, to see and admire them.)* You're proud of your body and you would like me to admire it. . . .

P: Yes . . . and to be sexually attracted to me. When I was sitting out in the waiting room, I had the fantasy of taking off all my clothes and then I would come in here and you would have all your clothes off too, and we would have sex on this analytic sofa! I still think about that even though we have talked about it so many times *(pause)*. . . . Today I had to go down to the university clinic. My wife wanted to go . . . but then she wanted to rush the doctor. . . . I told her I didn't want to rush the doctor. I wanted a full and complete evaluation. She acted miffed and it just upset me. . . .

N: She wanted to go and that felt supportive, but when she got anxious about her own appointment, it diminished the support and added to your anxiety . . .

P: Yes . . . I did want her support. You know, I always said that if I had someone's support, I could do anything . . . like a boss, or someone. . . . I needed my mom's support and I never really felt I had it. I remember I was in the bathtub one night with my brother. As my mom was drying me off, she said, "Tomorrow you will start first grade." I thought, "What?! I'm not ready for that! I don't want to go! I want to stay home with my mom!" I hadn't gone to kindergarten. She had never mentioned that I would go to school. It came as a complete surprise.

N: You've wanted and needed support and felt like you didn't get it from her and didn't get it from your wife this morning . . . and you need to be here with me in your analysis. . . . You don't want to be rushed or pushed out.

P: Yes . . . I fill . . . *(He means to say "feel" but says "fill.")* this void inside me. . . .

N: You fill the void with fantasies of being with women, now me. You'd like to be naked with me and have sex, and you would like me to see you and admire your body. . . . *(I continue to invite the erotized transference.)*

P: Yes . . . but I know that will never happen. *(It is getting near the end of the hour.)* I will try to fill the void, Nancy.

N: You said you would try to fill the void, as if you had to do that all by yourself . . . as if you didn't have me to help you with this. *(Here I am offering myself as a good object to be taken in.)*

P: *(His hands come up to his face. He struggles to hold back tears.)* I can't believe you said that! You are offering to help me with this . . . to fill up the void . . . this is so moving to me . . . (*after a pause*) . . . but I have to be careful . . . I have to remind myself that this is not an offer for sex . . . that is where my mind goes . . . but it is an offer for help . . . so I don't feel so scared and lonely . . .

N: Yes . . . that's right. . . .

Offering ourselves as objects for our patients' use

By the patient's projection and our introjection, we *actively seek and take in* beta experience, think about it, process it, and then return it to the heterogeneous patient – those patients who suffer from pre-Oedipal trauma and Oedipal/post-Oedipal conflicts. We do this by behavioral means and by interpretations. This is a variant of the normal mother/infant interpersonal communication.

In doing so, the patient's productions and suffering are contained. Ideally, the child also introjects the process of metabolizing affects himself and thereby introjects the dynamic of the container-contained (Bion, 1957, 1962), thereby developing his own internal thinking apparatus.

Mourning requires symbolic thinking, converting beta bits into alpha bits and then alpha functioning. It is through mourning that internal objects are created. Steiner said (1993, p. xii), "it is through the process of mourning that parts of the self are regained [in analysis]." Hanna Segal, in *Dream, Phantasy and Art* (1991, p. 40), writes, "A symbol is like a precipitate of the mourning for the object." If we pull from Kleinian and Bionian theory, we see that the baby does not have to think about the breast that is present, warm, soft, providing milk and comfort. But the absent breast, when the baby is hungry or when the breast is needed for comfort and reassurance, leaves the baby distressed, sometimes even falling apart, as if he were losing his mind. Likely all three of the cases presented here had that experience, especially M, whose infantile experiences emerged so clearly behaviorally and in her associations. The baby is searching in his mind/experience for the breast, and it is not there! It must be mourned and, in the mourning, the idea, the symbol appears of the "no-thing," the "no-breast," an absence. The symbol is a representation that can then become a part of an internal object. If the baby cannot gather up a memory and the idea of the "no-breast," his mind and experience will be chaotic, and a chronic inability to symbolize will leave him with psychotic foci.

The three cases presented in this chapter are what in Freud's time likely would have been considered *interminable, not fully treatable* cases. I believe he would have categorized them as such because he would have considered these patients' constitutional strengths, their id instincts, to be predominant and excessive. He would have felt they suffered from weaknesses of the ego, masochism, and so on.

All the cases presented herein suffered in Steiner's (1993) psychic retreat or the presence of a *gang* of repressed internalized bad object (experiences), a derivative of Fairbairn's theory that bad object experiences are repressed and become the anti-libidinal ego or internal saboteur that then sadistically tortures the patient. In these cases, the suffering caused by the internal saboteurs was manifest by loneliness, feelings of emptiness, severe anxiety, compulsivity, obsessions, and a sense of there not being a self and at other times experiencing a collapsed, psychotic mind.

All of the cases were also examples of Andre Green's (1972) *Dead Mother Complex*. They each had internal mothers whose alpha functioning, ability to symbolize, was weak or nearly absent, so that these patients did not sufficiently develop symbolic thinking. Instead L developed global embodied arousal as well as disorganized, hysterical thinking like Freud's Dora (1905); M developed obsessional thinking and compulsive behaviors; P filled his empty void with violence and sexuality because of insufficient symbolic thinking.

These cases were described to bring theory to life but also to give insight into the extended time needed to treat these patients; the care and thoughtfulness needed to properly manage the frame and the transferences; and the need to understand the countertransference and use it to understand the patient. Although it may seem as if I broke the frame in offering extended sessions and allowing the patient free rein of space, I believe I held a firm frame but held it gently. Perhaps what is most important is an analyst's capacity to hold the frame firmly intrapsychically, not just to prevent serious breaches and enactments but also to offer the patient the kind of well-grounded analytic mind needed to work through the painful early dynamic issues brought to analysis.

References

Ashbach, C. (2017). A reversible perspective: Who the subject? . . . Who the object? Presented at the International Psychotherapy Institute Master Speaker Seminar, Chevy Chase, MD, Fall.

Bakalar, N. (2017). The use of the self: When the patient is stuck, the therapist digs deeper. Presented at the International Psychotherapy Institute Master Speaker Seminar, Chevy Chase, MD, Spring.

Bion, W. R. (1957). Differentiation of the psychotic from the non-psychotic personalities. *The International Journal of Psychoanalysis*, 38: 266–275.

Bion, W. R. (1962). The psycho-analytic study of thinking. *The International Journal of Psychoanalysis*, 43: 306–310.

Bollas, C. (2013). *Catch Them before They Fall*. London: Routledge.

Fairbairn, W. R. D. (1944). Endopsychic structure considered in terms of object relationships. In *Psychoanalytic Studies of the Personality*. London: Routledge and Kegan Paul, 1952, pp. 82–135.

Fairbairn, W. R. D. (1963). Synopsis of object-relations theory of the personality. *The International Journal of Psychoanalysis*, 44: 224–225.

Ferro, A. (2003). Marcella: The transition from explosive sensoriality to the ability to think. *Psychoanalytic Quarterly*, 72: 183–200.

Freud, S. (1905). Fragment of an analysis of a case of hysteria (1905 (1901)). *Standard Edition,* 7: 1–122.

Freud, S. (1917). Introductory lectures on psycho-analysis, lecture XXVIII. *Standard Edition,* 16: 448–463.

Freud, S. (1933). New introductory lectures on psycho-analysis, lecture XXXIV. *Standard Edition*, 22: 136–157.

Freud, S. (1937). Analysis terminable and interminable. *Standard Edition*, 23: 209–253.

Green, A. (1972). The dead mother. In *On Private Madness*. London: Karnac, pp. 142–173.

Quinodoz, D. (2001). The psychoanalyst of the future: Wise enough to dare to be mad at times. *The International Journal of Psychoanalysis*, 82(2): 235–248.

Segal, H. (1991). *Dream, Phantasy and Art*. London: Routledge, p. 40.

Steiner, J. (1993). *Psychic Retreats: Pathological Organizations in Psychotic, Neurotic and Borderline Patients*. London: Routledge.

6 Can an ingroup be an internal object?

A case for a new construct

Ron B. Aviram

The concept of "ingroup" is not typically used in psychoanalysis. It is more familiar in social psychology, anthropology, and sociology. Similarly, "internal object" is not a concept that is utilized in those disciplines. Yet, if these two terms can be integrated across disciplines, the result of conceptually enriching each may become apparent. The limitation has persisted because one term refers to intergroup behavior, while the other term applies to unconscious processes in the context of interpersonal behavior. This chapter examines how identity groups are internalized and function unconsciously in the minds of individuals. It addresses the psychological transformation of the individual operating in an interpersonal context into an identity group member functioning in an intergroup context. The capacity to understand more about this complicated experience requires a construct that usefully explains how an identity group is internalized and thereby functions intrapsychically to influence behavior. The construct of a social object representation is discussed to clarify how an ingroup can be an internal object and how it can influence both self-experience and intergroup behavior.

"Ingroup" refers to an identity group in society to which an individual has an actual and psychological-emotional attachment. The ingroup contributes to our conception of ourselves, our self-concept. Related to the ingroup, the concept of "outgroups" refers to identity groups that we do not belong to and at times outgroups can be in conflict with our ingroup. It is clear that ingroups have a significant impact on human lives. In order to understand whether ingroups can become internal objects, we need to clarify what internal objects represent.

In this chapter, "internal object" refers to the internalization of an external object with which one has a significant relationship. Although there is no consensus about what constitutes an internal object across varying psychoanalytic models, most of the time when we speak about objects we are referring to other people. "Internal object" refers to the internalized representation of an affective connection between the self and an other (Kernberg, 1976). Importantly, it can also pertain to the relationship of the self with an animate or inanimate object, which is satisfying or unsatisfying (good or bad).

The pioneers of psychoanalysis had to formulate concepts that articulate what is happening when experiences of relationships are internalized and become dynamically influential in the course of a human life. Abraham (1911), Ferenczi (1909), and Freud (1917) introduced three constructs associated with internalization. Taken together, they describe psychic maturation of internalization processes. *Incorporation* and *introjection* are more primitive forms of internalization. In these two psychologically early forms of internalizing an external object, distinct self-other differentiation is not complete. These processes are building blocks for psychically associating with the external world. They provide a means for the self to take in or "internalize" experiential dimensions of the relationship with the object (initially the mothering person). As self-other differentiation develops, new experiences of relating can be internalized. The process of *identification* facilitates a more mature form of relationship with an object. Freud (1921) suggested that identification is "the earliest expression of an emotional tie with another person" (p. 105), at which point distinct self-other differentiation is present. This comment foreshadowed an object relations perspective in which the experience of oneself is interdependent with the object. Internal objects are important in clinical psychoanalysis because they provide a conceptual basis for understanding how external experience can be internalized, allowing the mind thereby to influence behavior, pathology in particular.

The concept of internal object relations was described by many theorists throughout the twentieth century, each having his or her particular emphasis (Director, 2018). (For a thorough overview of the evolution of ideas regarding internal objects see Ogden [1983].) The focus of this chapter is on an unconventional use of the concept of internal object. The emphasis will be on how large groups (specifically identity groups) influence the development of mind, perception of self and other, and, most important, groups of others. Fairbairn's (1952) ideas about internal objects are well suited for this purpose. A core tenet of Fairbairn's perspective is that libido is object seeking. In other words, individuals are oriented toward other people from the beginning. He believed that human motivation is oriented toward facilitating satisfying and cooperative relationships. However, given the inevitable imperfection of relating, he believed that we internalize the unsatisfying experiences of relationships with our first significant others (parental figures). This happens as a way to manage the anxiety aroused by dependence upon these unsatisfying but significant external others. The fact that these experiences are negative leads to their repression, and this establishes the first internal objects. Fairbairn's internal objects are completely dependent upon the behavior of the external object (individuals).

Internal objects are pathological in Fairbairn's unique metapsychology. This is logical if the definition of internal objects is that they are established through repression of "bad" experiences with external objects. Fairbairn did not see any reason for a satisfying relationship (a good object) to be repressed. Therefore, only bad objects, which cannot be tolerated consciously, are internalized and then repressed, becoming internal objects. The internal object is a defensive effort to deal with a frustrating and unsatisfying external object. Fairbairn suggested that at a very early time in development the infant establishes internal objects to make up for not having a satisfying external object (1952, p. 34). The self is dependent upon the external object from the beginning. From a developmental perspective, pathology is an outcome of what Fairbairn called infantile dependence persisting into adulthood. In this mode Fairbairn writes, "the object with which the individual is identified becomes equivalent to an incorporated object, or to put it in more arresting fashion, the object in which the individual is incorporated is incorporated in the individual" (1952, pp. 42–43). If this is true, it explains how a significant external object can have a place in the mind.

The self is unavoidably, to varying degrees, intertwined with external objects. When the inevitable unsatisfying aspects of a relationship upon which one is dependent become intolerable, they are repressed. This results in everyone having some degree of identification with an object, because parenting is never perfect. In other words, each person internalizes some aspects of the negative relationship with a significant other. People have internal objects because of the imperfection of human relations. This is why Fairbairn wrote that our identifications become our experience of ourselves (1952, p. 47). But, unlike Freud's use of identification as a tie to a differentiated object, for Fairbairn it is a basis for human interdependence. If this is an acceptable way to think about internal objects, could this suggest how ingroups (if they become significant objects upon which we depend) can have a place in the mind? And can it then explain how ingroups can thereby affect the way we behave and experience ourselves?

The first social group

In an early paper, Fairbairn (1935) articulated how the family context is associated with progressive "sociological" group formations. Extrapolating from there, we can say that this paper implies that an ingroup can have a place in the mind alongside internal objects that are associated with individuals of historical significance. Conceptually, the family is a holding environment for the individual caregivers. These significant individuals are the ones who become the original internal objects. Therefore, the family context influences these internal objects. In his paper, Fairbairn examined the evolution of social groups beginning with the family as the first social group. He described how the family is a fundamental component of subsequent larger groups such as clans, tribes, and nations. Fairbairn's description of the family as the first social group and how it is interrelated with larger social groups is an early psychoanalytic articulation of the formation of ingroups. Unacknowledged is the fact that the individuals who represent the first internalized objects in the mind operate within the larger group structure of the family. We tend to overlook the potential of the family and, possibly, the social groups that stem from it as internal objects (Aviram, 2014).

In dialectical fashion, individuals influence the family atmosphere, while the family atmosphere affects the individuals. Fairbairn believed that each person's loyalty to the family can be extended to identity groups, which become his or her ingroups. We can understand this to be an extension of his premise that libido is object seeking, now applied to important identity structures in society. So long as the groups do not seek to replace the family ties by demanding complete allegiance, he thought, individuals need and seek ingroup affiliations. Only pathological large groups like the fascist and communist movements in Fairbairn's time and, possibly, radical Islamic organizations such as ISIS in our time try to replace family bonds by demanding loyalty to the large group instead. They insist on becoming the individual's new family. These pathological ingroups try to eliminate the need for the family of origin. Fairbairn correctly predicted that those kinds of large groups would ultimately fail, because the family seems to be a core component of self that is rarely given up. In fact, it is likely that only the most internally fragile are willing to reject their association with the original family group. This perhaps offers a way to predict what will happen with the current destructive large groups in our epoch. Those familiar with Fairbairn's work will recognize the parallel between this description of the importance of the individual's tie to the family and his discovery that children do not relinquish ties with parents even if they are abusive. Here we have a parallel with another important concept in social psychology, called ingroup favoritism. It is a common finding that people favor their ingroup over outgroups (Hogg and Abrams, 1988). The internalized family provides a psychodynamic basis for the occurrence of this phenomenon in society. Most people do not seek out other families to replace their own. Fairbairn believed that the difficulty of rejecting poor caregivers was a reflection of the internalization and repression of the negative elements of the relationship. In adulthood, these internal "bad" objects continuously shape the course of life and perception of interpersonal relationships. They limit psychological growth and the potential for consciously engaged, mature interdependent relationships. In other words, unconscious processes, such as transference, shape relating.

Can a large group to which an individual belongs also become internalized in a way that can psychologically have an impact how that individual feels about himself or herself and influence perception and behavior? This would be similar to but not identical with how internal objects associated with individuals shape interpersonal relationships. If the family is the first social group, what happens to our early experience of this group? How is it represented in the mind? The influence of the family atmosphere is an important lasting emotional memory for most, if not all, individuals. The family, like a significant individual caregiver, is an early context upon which we are unconditionally dependent. The family can provide an additional layer of satisfaction and safety to the one offered by the interpersonal relationship with each caregiver. Both offer a context that meets physical and psychological needs. As the child and young adult emerge into the world beyond the atmosphere of the family, many of the identity groups that continue to meet the sometimes physical but certainly the emotional needs that began in the family also promote emotional well-being and can at times determine survivability.

At the same time, there are dissatisfactions with the family, in parallel to the individual caregivers. Clearly some family environments are emotionally and physically safer than others. Recall that Fairbairn believed that we internalize and repress "bad" or unsatisfying objects. If the family, the first social group, is "bad" and all families are to some extent, is it not possible that the family will also become a potential object for internalization? In that case, the bad aspects of the family are split off and repressed as bad objects. Fairbairn believed that our unconditional dependence upon the early environment is the ultimate cause of internalization and repression (Fairbairn, 1952, p. 66). Unconditional dependence is what makes "badness" intolerable in consciousness, in that survival is dependent upon this individual/family. Repression of the split-off bad aspects of the family allow one to continue to function in that context. As Fairbairn (1952) put it, "the sense of outer security resulting from this process of internalization is, however, liable to be seriously compromised by the resulting presence within [the person] of internalized bad objects. Outer security is thus purchased at the price of inner insecurity" (p. 65).

The social object representation

I have called this kind of internal object a *social object representation* (Aviram, 2005). The construct is needed in order to differentiate the social object representation from internal objects associated with interpersonal relationships of historical significance. It represents a place in the mind for the earliest experience of oneself as a family/group member. It lays the foundation in the mind for all subsequent associations with identity groups. The social object becomes the unconscious representation for our potential relationship with ingroups, society's extensions of early family experience, which, however, is not a substitute for the actual parents. These identity groups function as the external context through which to engage the dynamics associated with the human need to belong (Baumeister and Leary, 1995). This may be expressed by children when they feel insecure about their place in the family or how welcome they feel in peer groups. An example of this is the frequent report of having fantasized about being adopted. Another is a child "running away from home" by hiding in the bushes to see if someone will come to look for him. Later in development, teenagers wrestle with these feelings as they traverse high school territory with its large number of cliques.

Fairbairn's "endopsychic mind" was originally conceived to reflect interpersonal relations with individual caregivers. The first external object is the mother. The world is brought to the infant by this important first object. A developmental process unfolds with the first experiences dependent upon one other person. There has been precedent for considering that the object world can be multidimensional beyond a two-person relationship. For example, Scharff and Scharff (1987) introduced the representation of the internal couple that we carry of our parent's relationship. The internal representation of the parental couple influences subsequent marital relationships with needs for love and defenses against rejection.

In early life, the meaning of family also emerges to become the first social group. The family is greater than the sum of its parts. Experientially, the family offers something in addition to experiences provided by the mothering figures (and possibly siblings) in the infant's life. If the parents offer acceptance, the family can offer belonging. It is important to note that the family is not a parental substitution. This suggests that the family and subsequent large groups with which we affiliate can have independent effects on minds of individuals that cannot be anticipated as an outcome of interpersonal histories. If that is so, then we need a construct to represent the social groups with which we are all interdependent. I have commented before (Aviram, 2014), just as there is no baby without a mother (Winnicott, 1965), there is no adult without an identity group (nationality, race, religion, ethnicity, age cohort, profession, and so on).

Belonging is the experience of love that the group provides, alongside the caregiver's love, associated with acceptance and unconditional positive regard (Rogers, 1951). The dynamics of belonging play out on a continuum, from feeling like an outsider to being an insider. It is relatively common in psychoanalytic psychotherapy to discover the patient's underlying and long-standing experience of feeling like an outsider. This makes sense: if the maturational intent is to relate, then the struggle to belong takes shape in feeling like an outsider. Are feelings of being an outsider an indication of the "return of the badness" of the repressed social object? Initially, the dynamics of belonging occur within the family, but obviously it is relevant for identifications with one's clan, tribe, and nation – or any other identity group to which we develop an attachment as we go through life. To wish to belong is a common desire. It makes sense that if individuals struggle to establish meaningful, cooperative, and satisfying interpersonal relationships, at the group level they can struggle with similar feelings associated with belonging. If the family is as important as individual parents are, then libido continues to seek similar group affiliations. Regarding the social object, the seeking pertains to an atmosphere of belonging that was uniquely experienced with the family and is a continuation of our object-seeking nature.

A third internal object

In keeping with Fairbairn's notion of a dynamic endopsychic mind, the social object becomes a third "bad" object with which the libidinal and antilibidinal ego/selves engage under certain conditions. As an internal object that can influence our relationships with societal identity structures, the social object operates alongside Fairbairn's exciting and rejecting objects, which reflect interpersonal relations. Most of the time this third internal object is dormant. A majority of people do not participate in society with a constant awareness of their group identities. The social object representation, however, has the capacity to become a supraordinate internal object. What I mean by this is that any individual can be overwhelmed by societal conditions that are associated with identity groups. The most obvious examples are wars and societal stressors that manifest in prejudices, but it also operates in more common situations. For example, the social object may be activated when a police officer engages an African American in the United States. When young adults find their way into gangs, or cults, or the Boy Scouts, or armies, perhaps the social object is activated and influencing perceptions of oneself and others as group members. For sure, when sports fans from rival teams riot, it is unconsciously motivated; otherwise, why would such destructive behavior occur over such a trivial matter? Although appearing trivial, the significance of group belonging is the motivator. What about when men and women interact in a context with power differentials? At those moments, there is a psychological shift in which individuals perceive themselves and others as ingroup and outgroup members. For brief moments, they are not individuals; they are identity group members. Social psychologists have reported on this for a long time. They have found that when group identity is salient, individuals perceive themselves and others as group members rather than individuals (Hogg and Abrams, 1988).

Group membership and the social object

The implications for intergroup behavior are significant. When an individual psychologically transforms into a group member, the social object overrides the rejecting and exciting internal bad objects associated with interpersonal relations. When this occurs, there is a subtle experience of outsider or insider, inferior or superior, depending on the historical relationship one has had with group membership. The social object representation is the unconscious template for group belonging. At those moments, the social object influences behavior as a group member, rather than as an individual. For brief moments, and for some people for extended periods, relations with other people become intergroup relations. The social world has shifted into perceptions of group belonging and the unconscious need to establish safety. The threat can range from mild anxiety to annihilation anxiety. Anxiety initiates behavior that can be destructive in an effort to establish psychological safety. Individuals can be overwhelmed by social forces that turn them into group members (or create the perception of exclusion from the group). For example, during periods of economic hardship, otherwise tolerant people can become rejecting of outgroup members (immigrants, minorities, people with lower or higher socio-economic status). Stressful societal atmospheres can activate ingroup status as an avenue for emotional safety. To be part of a group offers safety in numbers, whereas the lone individual is more vulnerable. All individuals can be affected by these societal conditions. Therefore, all individuals are susceptible to the "return of bad social objects." Fairbairn explained, "an unconscious situation involving internalized bad objects is liable to be activated by any situation in outer reality conforming to a pattern which renders it emotionally significant in the light of the unconscious situation" (1952, p. 76). Furthermore, "when such bad objects are released, the world around the patient becomes peopled with devils which are too terrifying for him to face" (p. 69). Fairbairn dealt with the problem of a return of bad objects from the standpoint of interpersonal relationships. He suggested that when a person breaks down, it is a failure of repression that releases the bad object in the form of a malevolent mother or father.

When we encounter behavior connected to identity group status, it is not so much a malevolent mother or father emerging out of repression as much as activation of primitive associations with belonging. The implication of a failure of repression of the "bad social object" is that identity groups begin to represent survival in such a way that belonging is a matter of life and death. To be outside the ingroup is to be in a vulnerable situation, and the most extreme behaviors are likely to be associated with the earliest fearful perceptions of unconditional dependence upon the family. At that earliest period, as well as in adulthood, vulnerability and survival are interdependent with belonging to the family/ingroup.

The need to maintain an attachment to the family/ingroup becomes paramount when anxieties activate the repressed unconscious social object. Self-protective defenses begin to influence perception. This relies on the defense of splitting that simplifies the world. The axis of belonging that engages the continuum from being a lonely outsider to being a desperate insider will determine how splitting will operate. This defensive stance is maintained so firmly because, as Fairbairn put it, it is literally a matter of life and death (1952, p. 67). In a context of competing identity groups, individuals who manifest the dynamic of the insider are at higher risk for destructive intergroup behavior than the outsider. For the insider, the ingroup is used defensively to provide safety and self-esteem. Under more threatening conditions, how he or she treats the outgroup is a function of many variables and is especially dependent upon societal norms, deterrents, and ingroup leaders' messages about the outgroup. Societies have developed ways to contain the risks of this destructive process most of the time. The degree to which a person identifies with his or her ingroup is an outcome of several variables. If societal conditions are threatening (e.g., war), most people will be strongly identified with the ingroup/ nation. When conditions are less threatening in society, the influence of the unconscious will operate to determine the degree of identification with the ingroup. The person overidentified with his ingroup reflects libidinal needs at a group level that manifest in a feeling of superiority. In contrast, the outsider struggles with vulnerability of isolation but is often passive, looking on, feeling excluded or inferior.

Consider an example I observed of this in society. A Caucasian man stepped in front of a woman of color on a line for a rest room. The woman did not accept his slight and informed the man that she was waiting on the line, requesting that he return to his place behind her. He seemed to have made an assumption that she was not a customer in the shop because he told her that the rest room was only for customers. She explained that she would be buying something after she used the bathroom. At that point he increased his hostility and told her to "go back to where [she] came from." I am sure he did not mean "outside the store"! In that context, it was understandable that he was referring to some far-off native land. She understood that he was attacking her with prejudice. She remained composed and told him that he would be going after her, as she stepped in front of him and calmly held her place on line.

We can understand such incidents by recognizing that this man was overidentified with his ingroups of white, male, and American, implying that the woman was not an equal as an outgroup member. His behavior was dismissive of her as a person. At that moment, her social object was activated as a foreigner, a woman of color. Our hypothesis regarding this event is that the man was overidentified with an ingroup, which activated an entitled superiority in relation to the woman outgroup member. He perceived her not as an individual but rather as a member of an outgroup. The woman herself appeared to have maintained an optimal balance between being a group member and being an individual, all indicative of psychological health. The capacity to function effectively as both an individual and a member of a group even when ingroup status is activated is healthy. If this were not the case, it is likely that this event would have escalated as the two individuals became group members, each representing the outgroup for the other. When the threat becomes too great, optimal balance dissolves for most people.

The psychodynamics of the social object

A person within an optimal range balances autonomy as an individual with functional group belonging. This healthy balance permits the social object to function as a dormant third internal object, while the person participates in society with other individuals interpersonally. Balance of autonomy as an individual with functional ingroup attachments assists the overall functional wholeness of the self. This helps the group dimension of human life to enhance and strengthen one's existence. Individuals who fall beyond the outsider-to-insider optimal range, at the extremes of the Bell curve, manifest difficulties that show up in the way they feel about group belonging. For these individuals, the social object is activated in a way that overshadows internal objects of interpersonal relations (rejecting and exciting "bad" objects in Fairbairn's scheme).

Experientially, the outsider (beyond the optimal range) struggles with his or her perception of rejection from the group. These individuals can recognize feelings of resentment and jealousy. They may look at what others seem to have together or how happy they seem to be, and yet they do not feel that they can be part of the group. Outsiders feel fragile in society. They look on and perceive that other people feel connected with each other in a way that eludes them. If they do participate in a group it tends to offer a transient sense of belonging. Their group identity is precarious, and they do not feel secure in their experience of belonging. Such individuals are likely to come for psychotherapy when their sense of being outsiders becomes unbearable in the form of detachments from others. They then report an inability to form lasting relationships or a feeling that what they have is not good enough or their ongoing insecurity in trusting whether someone does or could love them. If you ask, they are likely to report that they have always felt like outsiders. Their family histories will indicate something about this experience. These individuals live out Fairbairn's recognition that internal bad objects provide external security at the cost of internal insecurity. They bring this into the world of social groups. They perceive the ingroups from which they are excluded as all good, while they themselves are bad.

The insiders (those outside the optimal range) tend to overidentify with the ingroup. These individuals need the group to feel secure. They probably have a history of seeking a variety of groups to shore up their self-esteem. The ingroup can play that role so long as it does not disappoint. The overzealous soldiers that Fairbairn (1943) wrote about who were sidelined and then had breakdowns represent this group. These are also the prejudiced individuals in a society. As a result of the overidentification with the ingroup, these individuals tend to perceive all others as either ingroup or outgroup members. They tend to function at a group level, rather than the interpersonal level. This manifests in idealization of the ingroup and disparagement and hate of the outgroup. The overidentification reveals the underlying pathology of the social object. For these individuals, the self and the ingroup have merged. These individuals try to reverse Fairbairn's notion about external security at the expense of internal insecurity. For the insider, a semblance of internal security is achieved with the merger of the self and ingroup. In this case, splitting operates to maintain the ingroup/self as all good and superior, thereby making them individually superior. This comes at the cost of external insecurity with outgroups that constantly feel threatening. These individuals are not likely to come to psychotherapy for their intergroup attitudes. However, addressing interpersonal crises with other ingroup members and enhancing personal self-worth can shift the overidentification with ingroups by initiating more secure autonomy as an individual.

Effects of psychotherapy on the social object

In an interpersonal relationship, which the psychotherapy context offers, the identity group is not often highlighted. In therapy, the two individuals form a bond that is interpersonal. That does not mean that the identity group dimension of the relationship is not noticed or talked about. Therapists can check with patients regarding historical experiences that pertain to belonging as a way to give voice to the part of mind associated with the social object.

The pathology of the social object is an aberration of our relational needs, expressed in terms of the need to belong that groups provide. It is built on the developmentally preceding interpersonal experiences one has had with caregivers. Even though individual pathology associated with the interpersonal world can be present, a pathology of group belonging can also affect the course of life. The social object implies that individuals seek affiliation with identity groups in similar ways to early family group experiences.

The good social object

Fairbairn was criticized for not making room in his endopsychic model for a good object to also be an internal object. His logic did not permit him to equate the two experiences in the unconscious. Repression was strictly for bad, intolerable experiences. This also made sense when considering that Fairbairn believed that infants are born whole with an unsplit, "pristine central ego." The infant is innately oriented to seek positive, cooperative, and satisfying relations with its external objects from the beginning. It implies that the infant starts life with a whole good object. It is only after the inevitable dissatisfactions become chronically experienced that repression of the split-off, intolerable rejecting or exciting but unsatisfying aspects of the relationship with the external object happens.

Fairbairn (1958) understood that the personal relationship with an analyst offers to correct distorted internalized relationships with bad objects. This anticipates the view that a relationship with a good object provides multiple new configurations within the self system (Skolnick, 2014). This implies that subsequent positive relationships can heal pathology and bring one closer to the original potential of the self that starts out whole and good before bad experiences occur. A new positive relationship with an analyst offers a working-through process and simultaneously provides a real relationship that does not have to be repressed. Instead, it is experiential and functions in both conscious and preconscious fashions. An outcome of the relationship with the good external object reinstates the original object-seeking potential that can operate anew with less unconscious negative influence. Patients engage external good objects in healthier ways, and that implies more consciousness. The internalized but not repressed aspects of our historical experiences with good objects, as well as new experiences, can also be thought of as becoming suffused throughout the personality, as J. D. Sutherland, a colleague of Fairbairn, commented (Personal Communication, D. Scharff).

All this applies to relations with identity groups. People are conscious of their identity group affiliations. The group's values contribute to self-esteem. Some individuals struggle with belonging and cannot integrate the ingroup as a good object. For others, the possibility of using the ingroup as a compensation for a fragile self is useful but promotes other difficulties with outgroups. In these cases, the ingroup functions as an external good object. For these individuals, identification with the ingroup tends to become an overidentification. In Fairbairn's terms, primary identification has eliminated any differentiation between the self and the large group, and this is an indication of pathology. The social object represents the repression of difficulties with group affiliation that began with the first social group, the family. If and when new and positive relationships are engaged, the potential to rebalance the capacity to function as a person and a group member simultaneously can be instated.

Conclusion

In an otherwise healthy individual, the ingroup functions alongside the family, and the family operates as a support for the individual who engages interpersonally with others. The healthy individual is able to interact with a diverse set of individuals with little attention to the large-group membership of the other. Identity groups are important resources for people in society, complementing their interpersonal relationships. They exist as unavoidable categories of identity that extend developmentally outward from the original family. Identity groups represent the group dimension of our innate object-seeking nature. They function alongside our interpersonal relations, rather than taking over as an object upon which the person is fully dependent. The social object that is a bad internal object functionally engages with the external identity group in a way that shows how the need to belong is intertwined with survival and growth. In the pathologies of social objects, individuals struggle with either feeling like outsiders or merging with ingroups as overcompensation for their need to belong. Most people function within an optimal range. However, societal conditions can activate the social object with preference for outsider or insider dynamics for all people.

References

Abraham, K. (1911). Notes on the psychoanalytical investigation and treatment of manic-depressive insanity and allied conditions. In K. Abraham (Ed.), *Selected Papers on Psychoanalysis*. London: Hogarth Mifflin, 1942, pp. 137–156.

Aviram, R. B. (2005). The social object and the pathology of prejudice. In J. S. Scharff and D. E. Scharff (Eds.), *The Legacy of Fairbairn and Sutherland*. New York: Routledge, pp. 227–236.

Aviram, R. B. (2014). The family is the first social group, followed by the clan, tribe, and nation. In G. S. Clark and D. E. Scharff (Eds.), *Fairbairn and the Object Relations Tradition*. London: Karnac, pp. 471–482.

Baumeister, R. F. and Leary, M. R. (1995). The need to belong: Desire for interpersonal attachments as a fundamental human motivation. *Psychological Bulletin*, 117(3): 497–529.

Director, L. (2018). Revisiting the psychoanalytic object: Introduction. *Psychoanalytic Dialogues*, 28(1): 1–11.

Fairbairn, W. R. D. (1935). On the sociological significance of communism. In *Psychoanalytic Studies of the Personality*. London: Routledge, pp. 223–246.

Fairbairn, W. R. D. (1943). The war neuroses: Their nature and significance. *British Journal of Medical Psychology*, 19: 327–341. In: *Psychoanalytic Studies of the Personality* (pp. 59–81). London: Tavistock, 1952.

Fairbairn, W. R. D. (1952). *Psychoanalytic Studies of the Personality*. London: Routledge.

Fairbairn, W. R. D. (1958). On the nature and aims of psycho-analytical treatment. *International Journal of Psychoanalysis*, 29: 374–385.

Ferenczi, S. (1909). Introjection and transference. In *Contributions to Psychoanalysis* (Ernest Jones, Trans.), 1916. Boston: Richard G. Gadger, pp. 30–80. (Original work published in 1909).

Freud, S. (1917). *Mourning and melancholia. S.E.*, Vol. 14. London: Hogarth Mifflin.

Freud, S. (1921). *Group Analysis and the Psychology of the Ego. S.E.*, Vol. 19. London: Hogarth Mifflin.

Hogg, M. A. and Abrams, D. (1988). *Social Identifications: A Psychology of Intergroup Relations and Group Processes*. London: Routledge.

Kernberg, O. F. (1976). *Object Relations Theory and Clinical Psychoanalysis*. New York: Jason Aronson.

Ogden, T. (1983). The concept of internal object relations. *International Journal of Psychoanalysis*, 64: 227–241.

Rogers, C. (1951). *Client-Centered Therapy: Its Current Practice, Implications, and Theory*. Boston: Houghton Mifflin.

Scharff, D. and Scharff, J. S. (1987). *Object Relations Family Therapy*. Northvale, NJ: Jason Aronson.

Skolnick, N. J. (2014). The analyst as good object: A Fairbairnian perspective. In G. S. Clark and D. E. Scharff (Eds.), *Fairbairn and the Object Relations Tradition*. London: Karnac, pp. 249–262.

Winnicott, D. W. (1965). *The Facilitating Environment and Maturational Processes*. New York: International University Press.

7 Beyond subject and object, or why object-usage is not a good idea

Juan Tubert-Oklander

Classical psychoanalysis has had an anti-environmental bias. There were some personal determinants of this on Freud's part, but also various psycho-social factors and many of his philosophical and epistemological assumptions led him to hope that the discipline he had created would become just another natural science. This led to a theory-building strategy based on an individual paradigm, the primacy of the past (which seemed to fit quite nicely with causal explanations), and the focus on the intrapsychic. There have been many attempts to transcend this bias, from both a relational and a social and political perspective, which led to the development of group analysis. There have been various attempts to integrate the individual and the collective perspectives, and I believe there is an urgent need for a new paradigm of the human being, developed along these lines, based on and transcending both psychoanalysis and group analysis.

Nonetheless, the very nature of Freud's discovery of the procedure he devised for the treatment of and inquiry into neurotic afflictions and the experiences that emerge from it was of quite a different nature from the impersonal objective facts that characterize the natural sciences. Although he never openly acknowledged it, his work was more akin to the humanities than to the reductionist natural science he had received from his teachers. Yet he was also aware that his subject matter was imposing on him something different from what he had intended. In his case story of Elizabeth von R., in *Studies on Hysteria* (Freud, 1895d), he writes the following caveat:

> I have not always been a psychotherapist. Like other neuropathologists, I was trained to employ local diagnoses and electro-prognosis, and it still strikes me myself as strange that the case histories I write should read like short stories and that, as one might say, *they lack the serious stamp of science*. I must console myself with the reflection that the nature of the subject is evidently responsible for this, rather than any preference of my own.
>
> (p. 160, italics added)

Hence, he was afraid of losing "the serious stamp of science," perhaps because he was afraid that his discoveries and ideas might be rejected by the scientific and academic establishments he so passionately yearned to be a part of. But this was also an expression of a deep split in his personality, between two roots of his spiritual development: the physicalist science that prevailed in his medical studies and the German Romanticism he had absorbed from his cultural background, particularly through Goethe (Tubert-Oklander, 2008, 2017a). In any case, this deep split has remained ingrained in the further developments of psychoanalysis, establishing a gap, perhaps a chasm, between the analytic practice and experience on one hand and the formal theories that purport to account for them on the other.

It is usually said that the real beginning of psychoanalysis was on September 1897, when Freud (Letter of September 21, 1897, in Masson [1985], pp. 264–267) abandoned his so-called seduction theory – which was really a theory of the traumatic effects of child abuse – and turned his attention from environmental stimuli to the exclusive study of intrapsychic processes. He had come to the conclusion that his patients' descriptions of sexual abuse in childhood had never happened: they were either delusions or lies. But, surprisingly enough, he did not leave a single note documenting a case that led him to such conclusion. This was most atypical for Freud, who was always meticulous in clinical research. Such lack of documentary evidence, plus the passionate reactions of Freud and his circle whenever someone – such as Ferenczi (1933) – tried to take a new look at the traumatic theory of neuroses he had summarily discarded, suggests that there were unconscious emotional motives behind his decision.

Freud's original theory of an environmental causation of psychopathology was quite subversive, and generated intense and violent rejection from both his colleagues and the learned public. The mere suggestion that parents and other adult caregivers could and often did abuse and do harm to the children under their care undermined the very basis of social authority. For, if parents and relatives could not be fully trusted, this distrust would surely also apply to nurses, teachers, doctors, priests, analysts, policemen, and government officers – that is, anybody who had helpless people as charges. No wonder such ideas generated widespread animosity and outrage among the young doctor's colleagues (Tubert-Oklander, 2016)! And the very same thing happened when Ferenczi (1933) read, in the 1932 Weisbaden Congress, his paper "Confusion of Tongues between the Adults and the Child," which posed a revamped version of the traumatic theory and his technical suggestions for the treatment of severely traumatized patients. But this time the indignant individuals who viciously demolished him with utter disqualification and slander were his fellow psychoanalysts and former friends and students.

However, beyond these psycho-social unconscious emotional aspects, there were also a number of assumptions, characteristic of Western thought in the modern era, that underlay the theoretical paradigm that Freud strove to construct with his metapsychology, which emphasized the primacy and centrality of the individual. These were (i) materialistic metaphysics; (ii) the Cartesian subject; (iii) deterministic positivism; (iv) neutral objectivism; and (v) rejection of teleology.

The *materialistic metaphysics* that underlies positivistic natural science and most of our everyday conception of the world conceives the universe as a vast space in which there are objects – called "matter" – and forces – called "energy." This is the Newtonian conception of the universe, to which Freud adhered. Indeed, his 1895 *Project* (Freud, 1950a), which set the bases for his future metapsychology, took as a starting point the attempt to apply the Newtonian schema to develop a theory of the mind. Consequently, if only matter and energy are "real," the only possible basis for mental processes is the individual organism, and "mind" turns out to be a mere epiphenomenon of brain function (Tubert-Oklander, 2016). This conception has been surpassed by modern developments in physics and biology and most certainly contradicts the essence of Freud's major contributions.

The *Cartesian subject*, conceived as an autonomous mental entity, capable of thought, perception, and volition and neatly separated from the world of "objects" and from the body, came as an expression of the ethos of the bourgeoisie that emerged after the Renaissance. Up to that point, the only way to have access to riches, power, and prestige was through being born into the aristocracy, but now major merchants and businessmen could attain them by their own efforts. This fostered the belief that the individual was solely responsible for his destiny, in sharp contrast with the primacy of social structure in the Middle Ages. Even though Freud's discoveries and ideas undermined the alleged autonomy of the conscious subject, he still adhered to the centrality of the individual as the locus and starting point of all mental processes. This is particularly clear in the following quotation from "Instincts and Their Vicissitudes" (1915c):

> Let us imagine ourselves in the situation of an almost entirely helpless living organism, as yet unorientated in the world, which is receiving stimuli in its nervous substance. This organism will very soon be in a position to make a first distinction and a first orientation. On the one hand, it will be aware of stimuli which can be avoided by muscular action (flight); these it ascribes to an external world. On the other hand, it will also be aware of stimuli against which such action is of no avail and whose character of constant pressure persists in spite of it; these stimuli are the signs of an internal world, the evidence of instinctual needs. The perceptual substance of the living organism will thus have found in the efficacy of its muscular activity a basis for distinguishing between an "outside" and an "inside."
>
> (p. 119, italics added)
>
> The antithesis ego – non-ego (external), i.e. subject – object, is, as we have already said . . ., thrust upon the individual organism at an early stage, by the experience that it can silence external stimuli by means of muscular action but is defenceless against instinctual stimuli. *This antithesis remains, above all, sovereign in our intellectual activity and creates for research the basic situation which no efforts can alter.*
>
> (p. 134, italics added)

So, in the beginning was the individual, "an almost entirely helpless living organism," trying to discover the world, and the subject-object differentiation is an absolute fact, an antithesis that "remains, above all, sovereign in our intellectual activity and creates for research the basic situation which no efforts can alter." In other words, this is an assumption, a part of his *Weltanschauung*, which is previous to any psychoanalytic inquiry and inherently contradictory to the alternative assumption of a primary and essential social nature of the human being (Hernández Hernández, 2010; Hernández-Tubert, 2009).

By *deterministic positivism*, I refer to a certain view of science that prevailed in the nineteenth century (the period during which Freud was reared and had his scientific education) and that posited that everything that happens is determined by the strict laws of causality, so that an immensely powerful mind that had all the information about the relevant facts and the immutable laws of science (Laplace's Demon) would be able to predict all future events. In such a view, which has been refuted by the new developments of physics during the past century, the universe is conceived as a gigantic piece of clockwork, in which every possible move is determined by its structure and the initial conditions. This is clearly incompatible with a treatment such as psychoanalysis, which affirms that making conscious the unconscious determinants of a person's behavior can free the person from the chains of repetition and predictability that we call "psychopathology." Nonetheless, Freud firmly adhered to a belief in universal determinism, as can be seen in the following quotation from his *Introductory Lectures* (Freud, 1915–16):

> What does [it mean when someone speaks of "chance events"]? Is he maintaining that there are occurrences, however small, which drop out of the universal concatenation of events – occurrences which might just as well not happen as happen? If anyone makes a breach of this kind in the determinism of natural events at a single point, it means that he has thrown overboard the whole *Weltanschauung* of science. Even the *Weltanschauung* of religion, we may remind him, behaves much more consistently, since it gives an explicit assurance that no sparrow falls from the roof without God's special will.
>
> (p. 28)

One can only wonder what Freud would have thought of Heisenberg's principle of uncertainty and other developments in quantum theory or of Gödel's incompleteness theorems, which undermined the belief in predictability in physics and consistency in logic and mathematics!

Neutral objectivism implies that it is both possible and mandatory for a scientific observer to exclude himself from his descriptions so as to avoid contaminating his descriptions with his own subjectivity. An "objective" description is one that includes only data from the object under study and none from the observer who makes the description. In other words, it is a description of some state of affairs as if the observer were not there at all. But this is utterly at odds with contemporary developments in physics, biology, psychology, and most certainly psychoanalysis, which show that there is no way in which the observer's influence may not be a part of the phenomenon being observed. This is the gist of field theories, particularly of psychoanalytic field theories (Baranger and Baranger, 1961–62, 2008, 2009; Stern, 2013a, 2013b; Tubert-Oklander, 2007, 2017b), in which the observer is always a part of the field of observation.

The *rejection of teleology* has been an essential part of the scientific credo for a long time. Just as causal explanations account for a present event in terms of past events, teleological explanations do it in terms of some future state of affairs that is conceived as an aim or goal. This led to a discrediting of teleology, which was associated with religion and mysticism, since it seemed to imply an underlying intelligent intention or purpose, instead of the mechanics of an invariable chain of causation. Such an approach works quite well when dealing with the world of inanimate objects but inevitably fails when one is trying to account for the behavior of living beings in general and human beings in particular (Bateson, 1972), which always includes an intention.

Nevertheless, Freud's clinical method, with its emphasis on *meaning*, necessarily implies an underlying *intention*. This is the *principle of intentionality*, which the young Freud received from his teacher of philosophy Franz Brentano. It asserts that all psychic acts have an intention, that is, they tend to something – existent or inexistent, psychical or material – and this implies a relationship. Such teachings had an impact not only on Freud's psychoanalysis but also on Husserl's phenomenology.

The fact that Freud never mentions Brentano in his published writings is quite striking, particularly since Freud's letters of the time to his friend Edward Silberstein (Boehlich, 1990) show the profound impact that his teacher's thought and personality had had on him. Freud sought a personal relationship with Brentano and even considered entering the Faculty of Philosophy; on finding that it was not possible to study two careers at the same time, he still intended to do a doctorate in philosophy after completing his medical studies (Domenjo, 2000). So why this flagrant omission of Brentano's name? It may have to do with Freud's rejection of his teacher's theism. Be that as it may, this ablation of the memory of a person who had had a momentous influence on him, plus his later disparaging comments on philosophy, suggests that the youngster must have suffered a major disillusionment.

The case is that not only did Freud receive from Brentano the concepts of *representation* and *affect*, but "he also found in this author that which is intrinsically psychic in the *relationship between subject and object*, which Brentano calls *intention*" (Domenjo, 2000, p. 113). As this implied a teleological view of mental acts, Freud sought to reduce it to a causal (biological) explanation, and this he found in his theory of instinctual drives (Freud, 1915c), which to my mind does not really solve the problem.

All these assumptions upheld the individualistic paradigm, which reigned unchallenged in his metapsychology. But there was an alternative view of the human condition, one that had existed since classical Greek philosophy. While Plato's theory was based on the individual, Aristotle affirmed the essentially social nature of the human being. And the Aristotelean view had a much greater affinity to Freud's clinical discoveries and to the analytic experience. It is also worth noticing that he attended two courses on Aristotle taught by Brentano. Such a view underlay the relational tradition of psychoanalysis, from Sándor Ferenczi, through the authors of the British Independent Group (Fairbairn, Balint, Winnicott,

Rycroft, Milner, Little, Guntrip, Sutherland, and many others) and Interpersonal Psychoanalysis, up to contemporary Self Psychology, Intersubjective Theory, and Relational Psychoanalysis (Guntrip, 1961; Greenberg and Mitchell, 1983; Kohon, 1986; Aron, 1996; Clarke and Scharff, 2014; Tubert-Oklander, 2014a, 2018).

Although these relational perspectives took into account the relationships with other human beings, implicitly including relations with collective entities such as groups, communities, institutions, and society at large, they still viewed these relationships from the perspective of the individual. Of course, this was to be expected, since the psychoanalytic experience emerged from and was explored through the bi-personal device of clinical psychoanalysis. But there was still another way, which also derived from the inquiry of the unconscious aspect of human life inaugurated by Freud but did it by means of a different setting and technical device. This was what became known as *group analysis*.

Group analysis is something quite different from psychoanalytic group psychotherapy. The latter consists in applying the well-established theories and techniques of bi-personal psychoanalysis to the treatment of patients in groups. Group analysis, on the contrary, is the analytic inquiry of the shared experience people have in groups, whether therapeutic or non-therapeutic; small, medium, or large; natural groups or stranger groups. The group analyst does not just apply pre-existent psychoanalytic knowledge, ideas, or techniques but approaches the group with an analytic attitude and develops new interpretations and theories to account for the group-analytic experience in the same way psychoanalysts ever since Freud have done with the psychoanalytic experience derived from the bi-personal psychoanalytic situation. In doing so, group analysis has had to rely upon and lean on the contributions of the social sciences and the humanities, just as Freud did with biology and other natural sciences. But in both cases, the gist of their research is to be found in the analytic experience itself.

Group analysis emerged, independently and simultaneously, in two far-away places: in England. with S. H. Foulkes (1948, 1964, 1975), and in Argentina, with Enrique Pichon-Rivière (1971, 1979; Tubert-Oklander and Hernández de Tubert, 2004; Losso, de Setton and Scharff, 2017). Even though it was Foulkes who coined the term "group analysis" and although the name usually refers to the school he founded, while Pichon-Rivière called his own approach "operative groups," I strongly feel that the similarities between their respective thinking and practices far outweigh their minor differences, so that they may be viewed as two forms of a same praxis (I use this term to refer to a dialectical process of putting theories into practice and theorizing the experiences derived from practice).

But even though group analysis strove to transcend the limitations imposed by the individualistic paradigm, most group analysts remained fettered by their allegiance to some theory of the personality, which they used to understand the pathology and dynamics of the individual members of their groups. Hence, a Freudian psychotherapist would carry out a Freudian group analysis, a Jungian would do Jungian group analysis, and so on. And, indeed, we need to find a way of viewing, understanding, and dealing with intra-personal, inter-personal, and trans-personal phenomena and experiences, without being split between diverse theories, based on different assumptions. And this requires the development of a new paradigm of the human being (Hernández-Tubert, 2011; Tubert-Oklander, 2017a).

Such a paradigm implies a conscious inquiry and revision of many of the underlying assumptions that are the bases of all our thinking, feeling, and acting – in other words, our *Weltanschauung* (conception of the world) and *Lebensanschauung* (conception of life). These conceptions constitute a psychological structure, which is largely unconscious and stems from the unconscious aspects of social life and is internalized from all our relations, starting with the very first introjections and reinforced by all our later interpersonal and social experiences. This accounts for the almost unquestionable certainty with which we uphold these assumptions, which we do not usually perceive as being assumptions at all but only as "the way things are" (Hernández Hernández, 2010; Hernández-Tubert, 2009).

Of course, trying to develop a new paradigm of the human being in order to transcend the limitations of the old paradigm requires that the implicit assumptions of the latter be made explicit so that their implications can be sorted out and duly criticized. This is an arduous work, since it implies not only an epistemological criticism of the underlying bases of our theories and practices but also an analytic work of interpretation and working through of the powerful emotional forces and social injunctions that oppose the disclosure and questioning of these assumptions.

In our discipline, the task is even harder because the analytic identity is based on a frequently non-analyzed transference with Freud and other founding fathers or mothers of the analytic tradition into which the would-be analyst is being initiated (Tubert-Oklander, 2014b). Hence, our frequent unsolvable theoretical discussions with other colleagues who espouse views different from our own are not really about theory but instead are about our underlying world views and emotional allegiances to ideal objects (Hernández Hernández, 2010; Hernández-Tubert, 2000, 2015).

As I posed at the beginning of this chapter, Freud´s passionate desire to be a great scientist was in conflict with the real nature of the intellectual, relational, and social revolution he had initiated when he created psychoanalysis. He insisted over and over again that psychoanalysis should become a natural science and ignored the fact that his creation was bound to demolish the very bases of that positivistic science that he firmly believed to be the only possible way to reliable knowledge (Freud, 1933a). This obviously created a split in him, which is to be found all through his written work and which has been unconsciously transmitted to the subsequent generations of analysts, who also had to deal with their idealized and often ambivalent transference relation with their forefather.

This is a most complex issue, which deserves a more extensive study. At the moment, I wish to illustrate the form in which these unconscious conflicts were dealt by a well-acknowledged psychoanalytic pioneer and innovator, Donald Woods Winnicott, and how they limited the scope of his contributions. This is a major example of the contradictions and conflicts that emerge when we try to revise our deeply rooted beliefs.

Winnicott's contribution to the development of psychoanalysis was truly revolutionary, but he did not conceive of his work that way. He frequently declared in his writings that he had nothing to add to the generally accepted theory and then expounded his ideas on what he apparently viewed as a minor detail, without appearing to notice that they were truly incompatible with some major aspects of Freudian theory. One clear instance of this is his reformulation of the psychoanalytic theory of motivation (Tubert-Oklander, 2017c).

In his classical paper "Metapsychological and Clinical Aspects of Regression within the Psycho-analytical Set-up" (1955), he introduces a distinction between "wishes" and "needs." A wish seeks gratification, and, if this is not found, the result is frustration. A need is neither gratified nor frustrated; it is either met or not, and if it is not responded to, "the result is not anger, only a reproduction of the environmental failure situation which stopped the processes of self growth" (p. 22). Later, in "The Capacity to Be Alone" (Winnicott, 1958), he introduces the concept of an *ego-relatedness*, quite different from an *id-relationship*, to refer to a non-instinctual bond between mother and child or between patient and analyst. He sees this bond as most important, as he considers it to be "the stuff out of which friendship is made" and which "may turn out to be the matrix of transference" (p. 418).

In 1960, he comes back to this subject, in "Ego Distortion in Terms of True and False Self." There he explicitly differentiates "ego-needs" from "id-needs." Id-needs are the instinctual wishes – sexual or aggressive – of drive theory. They are organic tensions that tend to a pleasurable discharge, which we call "gratification." When this is lacking, there is an experience of unpleasure, which breeds irritation and anger, called "frustration." Ego-needs, on the other hand, require a personal, loving, empathic, validating, and understanding response from another human being. These needs are neither gratified nor frustrated, since they have nothing to do with pleasure or displeasure. When they are met, the person's experience is not pleasure but a feeling of harmony and well-being, a sense that everything is as it should be; when they are not, the inner response is not unpleasure but a feeling of futility, hopelessness, and lack of meaning.

Winnicott was obviously introducing a radical change in the psychoanalytic theory of motivation, one that replaced Freud's purely functional biological concepts with a theory of personal relations. We could now say that the theory of drives belonged to Martin Buber's (1923) *I-It* world, while Winnicott's relational proposal was clearly placed in the *I-Thou* domain. Hence, it is quite surprising that his conclusion, at the end of the paper, is that these concepts should be "able to have an important effect on psycho-analytic work [but] as far as I can see it involves no important change in basic theory" (Winnicott, 1960, p. 152).

How is it possible that Winnicott failed to see the full import of his innovative ideas? Greenberg and Mitchell (1983) believed that this was a strategic move, intended to somehow disguise the implications of what he was saying and avoid conflict with his professional community. I do not think this to be the case. Winnicott was an original thinker, and he was quite adamant about his need to think and understand things in his own words and language, not in those of someone else (Rodman, 1987). But he also had a positive idealized transference with Freud and a yearning to belong to the tradition inaugurated by him. How was he to reconcile these seemingly incompatible needs? I believe he did it by means of a splitting, quite similar to the split in Freud between the practice he had created, focused on inner experience and meaning, and his passionate wish to turn it into a natural positivistic science.

This unconscious maneuver was helped by the fact that Winnicott rejected systematic thinking and grand formal reconstructions of thought. His own thinking was more fluid and dialectical. So he did have a tendency to avoid reading abstract theory. His feelings toward Freud were quite ambivalent: on one hand he loved and admired him, but on the other he was rebellious toward this overpowering father figure, and this led him to reject reading metapsychology. Consequently, he was free to use the regular psychoanalytical vocabulary in new and unexpected ways. But he also felt guilty about it. Thus, he wrote, in a letter to Clifford M. Scott of December 26, 1956, quoted by Brett Kahr in *D. W. Winnicott: A Biographical Portrait*, during his first term of office as president of the British Psycho-Analytical Society,

> I feel odd when in the president's chair because I don't know *my Freud* in the way a president should do; yet I do find I have Freud in my bones.
>
> (Winnicott, 1956, quoted in Kahr, 1996, p. 70)

"Having Freud in my bones" obviously refers to a deep identification, while "knowing my Freud" as a requisite for being a president suggests that the Society is an institution devoted to the preservation of the words and the idealized image of its founding father. How could he, in view of such deep-rooted feelings, acknowledge that he was actually discarding some of the basic axioms of the latter's theories?

Indeed, when he and Masud Khan wrote a review of Fairbairn's 1952 book *Psychoanalytic Studies of the Personality* (Winnicott and Khan, 1953), they, in spite of writing a very positive valuation, took exception to the fact that the author rejected and proposed a theoretical alternative to some of Freud's fundamental assumptions. Their main argument, which clearly showed some irritation, was as follows:

> A reviewer is in a less fortunate position than an ordinary reader, since Fairbairn makes a definite claim, and it must be this claim that gets the appraisal and the criticism. *The claim is that Fairbairn's theory supplants that of Freud. If Fairbairn is right, then we teach Fairbairn and not Freud to our students.* If one could escape from this claim one could enjoy the writings of an analyst who challenges everything, and who puts clinical evidence before accepted theory, and who is no worshipper at a shrine. But the claim is there.
>
> (p. 329, my italics)

Of course, this criticism was not valid, since it relied on the fallacy called the argument *ad verecundum* – resorting to authority: "this cannot be so because it contradicts the sayings of a most prestigious author" (Tubert-Oklander, 2018). But it is even more surprising when we consider that Fairbairn's most objectionable assertion was that the main motivation behind human experience, thought, and behavior is the search for the object – that is, relationship – and not the search for pleasure. This he posed in the following terms:

> Libido is primarily object-seeking (rather than pleasure-seeking, as in the classic theory), and that it is to disturbances in the object-relationships of the developing ego that we must look for the ultimate origin of all psychopathological conditions.
>
> (Fairbairn, 1944, p. 82)

This was precisely the very same idea Winnicott had been working on for some time and that he developed in the papers of 1955, 1958, and 1960, quoted earlier. It was to become the theoretical foundation of the British Independent Group's Object Relations Theory. But Winnicott never wrote it as a disagreement with Freud. Indeed, the only issue on which he openly disagreed with his master was Freud's concept of the "death instinct," as he wrote in the following quotation:

> I have never been able to follow anyone else, not even Freud. But Freud was easy to criticize, because he was always critical of himself. For instance, I simply cannot find value in his idea of a Death Instinct.
>
> (Winnicott, 1962, p. 171)

It is true that he was never able to follow or use anyone else's language, as he was too intent on thinking things through in his own words. But it was also true that he had deep feelings of love, gratitude, admiration, and even awe toward Freud. Hence, what both he and Khan criticized in Fairbairn was not his original ideas, which were akin to theirs, but the fact that he openly acknowledged that they were incompatible with some of the basic tenets of Freudian theory. It must be said, to their credit, that both of them later recanted what they had written, recognizing that they had not really understood Fairbairn's ideas at that time (Clarke, 2014, p. 303).

These are some of the emotional factors that oppose the possibility of a major revision of the generally accepted theories. But there are other, subtler pressures that are much more difficult to perceive, identify, and think through. These have to do with the general assumptions about reality, knowledge, and the human condition that constitute our *Weltanschauung*. And these usually persist under the arguments of even the most revolutionary thinkers, as we have seen in the case of Freud. I shall now examine, as a clear example of this, Winnicott' s (1969) conception of the use of the object.

Donald Winnicott read the paper called "The Use of an Object" (Winnicott, 1969) to the New York Psychoanalytic Society on November 12, 1968. He was sternly criticized by the three official discussants (Edith Jacobson, Samuel Ritvo, and Bernard Fine), who took all the allotted time, so that there was no space for a discussion with the very large audience. They obviously did not understand or accept his arguments and his idiosyncratic use of language, and, although the transcripts of the session describe "a spirited intellectual exchange without signs of personal animosity or rancor" (Goldman, 1993, p. 216), there is also some evidence that the reaction to Winnicott's paper was quite violent:

> [S]ome participants in the meeting clearly recall an atmosphere of profound intolerance toward Winnicott's originality (Annie Bergman, personal communication, June 16, 1992). In the aftermath of the formal presentation, one participant noticed Winnicott to be visibly shaken and overheard him commenting that he now understood better why America was in Vietnam (Steven Ellman, personal communication, May 15, 1992).
>
> (p. 216)

Be that as it may, Winnicott, who had already come to the session feeling ill, developed pulmonary edema while still in New York and had to be hospitalized in a cardiac care unit for several weeks. So, there are some grounds for the interpretation that the fact that he had not been able to convey an idea that was obviously very important to him and had instead received a hostile response had at least contributed to the aggravation of his medical condition (Goldman, 1993).

But what had Winnicott said in his presentation? In a nutshell, his argument was as follows. For him, there was a basic distinction between what he called "object-relating" and "object-usage." As he had already written in many previous articles, he believed that the starting point for the baby is a state of non-discrimination, in which the infant is not aware of the existence of the mother. This determines an "absolute dependence [since] the infant has no means of awareness of maternal provision" (Winnicott, 1963, p. 87). At this stage, the object has become vitally and emotionally significant for the child but is not yet perceived as existent in its own right. This he calls "object-relating." If the mother is good-enough, her ministrations come more or less at the time in which the baby's need of her arises and the infant evokes the memory of previous encounters with her. This creates for the infant the illusion that he has created the object with his desire. This is what Freud (1900a) conceived as a hallucination of the memory of the experience of satisfaction, but Winnicott saw it not as a hallucination but as an *illusion* – a perception of something that is really there, but with an added subjective meaning. Such an object, perceived as if it were created by the child, he called a "subjective object," and this relation he called "object-relating."

But this illusion, which determines a normal, desirable, and phase-adequate feeling of omnipotence in the baby, is bound to collapse sooner or later, particularly when the mother emerges from her regressive state of "primary maternal preoccupation" (Winnicott, 1963) and starts recover her life, The baby reacts to this with a bout of destructive hate that in his present state of omnipotence should have annihilated the mother, but, to the infant's surprise, she survives it and is still there. This is a breakdown of the previous omnipotence and the beginning of the belief in an outside world, since it brings the first inkling that Mother really exists as a separate object. It is the end of the subjective object and the birth of the real object, which the child is now able to use, because it is real and full of unsuspected qualities to be discovered and enjoyed. Hence, object-relating is replaced by object-usage.

Winnicott (1969) describes this in the following terms:

> The subject can now use the object that has survived. It is important to note that it is not only that the subject destroys the object because the object is placed outside the area of omnipotent control. It is equally significant to state this the other way round and to say that it is the destruction of the object that places the object outside the area of the subject's omnipotent control. In these ways the object develops its own autonomy and life, and (if it survives) contributes in to the subject, according to its own properties.
>
> In other words, because of the survival of the object, the subject may now have started to live a life in the world of objects, and so the subject stands to gain immeasurably; but the price has to be paid in acceptance of the ongoing destruction in unconscious fantasy relative to object-relating.
>
> (p. 713)

The very same thing happens in the psychoanalytic treatment of severely traumatized patients: the patient destroys the analyst and the analyst survives, thus becoming a real person to him.

This was a revolutionary statement, which was understandably misunderstood and rejected by his three New York discussants. So, why do I say that this paper shows, at one and the same time, his deep theoretical innovations and his subservience to the old individualistic paradigm? Winnicott had been striving, during his whole career, to develop a view of psychoanalysis in terms of personal relations, which should have led him to a fully intersubjective theory and practice. But both his allegiance to Freud and the fact that he was a medical doctor and had great respect for natural science shackled him to the objectivistic conception upheld by science, philosophy, and common sense. This is shown by the terms he chose.

First, we have the unfortunate use, which is generalized in psychoanalytic discourse, of the abstract terms "subject" and "object," which conceals the fact that we are talking about relations between real living persons, not mere acts of perception or use of things. Such language is clearly positioned in the I-It construction of the world and not in the I-Thou one (Buber, 1923).

Then we have the fact that Winnicott, as well as most of the writers of the Independent object-relations tradition, were striving to include the "real other" in the understanding of the subject – whether a child or a patient – but did so almost exclusively from the standpoint of the individual. In Winnicott's theories, both Mother and the analyst have a major impact on the human being who is under their care, *but only as functional objects*. Winnicott's "mother" is either "good-enough" or "not-good-enough" in fulfilling her child-care functions, but nothing is said of her as a person, her subjectivity, her fears, her wishes, her dreams, her feelings, and the impact they have on her child. So, he stopped short of entering the intersubjective domain. The same is true for the patient-analyst relation. In this he strictly adhered to the medical and psychoanalytical tradition of keeping an absolute asymmetry in therapeutic relations. He could have found some elements in Sándor Ferenczi to aid him in revising such overpowering assumptions, but Winnicott also rejected reading Ferenczi. Indeed, he once said that he "was reluctant to read the works of Ferenczi, lest he discover that he had actually stolen ideas from him" (F. Robert Rodman, personal communication to Dodi Goldman [1993], p. 5). Besides, Ferenczi's 1932 *Clinical Diary* (Ferenczi, 1985), which described his experiments in mutual analysis, was only published in French in 1985 and in English in 1988.

Third, there is the underlying assumption, which Freud seems to have derived from Darwin's evolutionary theory (Frank J. Sulloway, interviewed by Rudnytsky [2000], pp. 137–209) and Haeckel's biogenetic law (Peter J. Swales, interviewed by Rudnytsky [2000], pp. 275–345), that human development follows a linear course, from the more primitive and undifferentiated stages to the more mature and normal ones. In such a view, "normal" means the usual mental state of a waking cultured adult male in our present society, and other forms of mental organization, such as those of children, women, mental patients, the lower classes, and the "primitives" – that is, non-European – are to be considered underdeveloped or even pathological. Freud argued, in *Civilization and Its Discontents* (1930a), that an undifferentiated phase, which he called "oceanic feeling," was a most primitive state of mind, characteristic of the baby, which should be completely overcome during normal development, remaining active in adulthood only in pathological cases, and that it had nothing to offer to normal psychic functioning. And this is the generally accepted version of orthodox psychoanalysis. But the idea that such an organization persists as an alternative form of experience during the whole lifetime is what allows us to transcend the abyss that the subject-object differentiation introduces between persons in the individualistic paradigm. Winnicott, who was striving to develop a relational theory, was nonetheless tied to this traditional view of existence and conceived personality development as a progression "from dependence to independence" (1963) and from subjectivity to objectivity (1969), and this prevented him from taking his nascent relational practice and theory to its logical conclusions (Tubert-Oklander, 2014c).

Finally, there is the very concept of "object use." The term "use," in common parlance, has connotations of exploitation and abuse. I know this is not what Winnicott meant; what he was trying to say is that a real other is much more satisfactory than an invented object that emerges from the baby's omnipotence. But why did he choose this unfortunate term? I believe that he was influenced by Freud's assumption, which is a dogma of faith in our current social organization derived from the Industrial Revolution, that the human being is essentially selfish and strives only for the satisfaction of his needs and wishes, as Freud clearly said in *Civilization and Its Discontents* (1930a) when he wrote that "we assume quite generally that the motive force of all human activities is a striving toward the two confluent goals of utility and a yield of pleasure" (p. 95). Winnicott, who had witnessed, as a pediatrician, thousands of mother-child interactions, knew better than that, since he had seen how babies, from the very beginning, showed expressions of concern and care for their adult caretakers. In the same vein, he acknowledged and accepted, in his clinical practice, his patients' expression of love, care, and concern for their analyst. But nonetheless, he still insisted in his belief in the baby's "ruthlessness" (Guntrip, 1975).

I hope that this brief study of Winnicott's contradictions may serve to illustrate the formidable and sometimes insurmountable difficulties we have to face when we attempt to identify, question, and revise the set of implicit and frequently unconscious assumptions that underlie our cherished theories and practices. But there is, nonetheless, a most urgent need for us to do so, in order to contribute to the development of the new paradigm of human life we so sorely need. Such a paradigm cannot emerge only from psychoanalysis, since it is being constructed from many sources in science, the humanities, art, religion, politics, and society, but we should do our best effort to ensure that psychoanalysis have a place in this transcendental change for humankind (Tubert-Oklander, 2019).

References

Aron, L. (1996). *A Meeting of Minds: Mutuality in Psychoanalysis*. Hillsdale, NJ: Analytic Press.

Baranger, M. and Baranger, W. (1961–1962). La situación analítica como campo dinámico [The analytic situation as a dynamic field]. *Revista Uruguaya de Psicoanálisis*, 4(1): 3–54. [English translation published in 2008.]

Baranger M. and Baranger, W. (2008). The analytic situation as a dynamic field. *International Journal of Psycho-Analysis*, 89: 795–826. [Original Spanish publication in 1961–1962.]

Baranger M. and Baranger W. (2009). *The Work of Confluence: Listening and Interpreting in the Psychoanalytic Field* (L. Glocer Fiorini, Ed.). London: International Psychoanalytic Association/Karnac.

Bateson, G. (1972). *Steps to an Ecology of Mind*. New York: Ballantine.

Boehlich, W. (1990). *The Letters of Sigmund Freud to Eduard Silberstein 1871–1881*. Cambridge, MA: Harvard University Press.

Buber, M. (1923). *I and Thou* (R. G. Smith, Trans.). Edinburgh: T. & T. Clark, 1937.

Clarke, G. S. (2014). John Padel's contribution to an understanding of Fairbairn's object relations theory. In G. S. Clarke and D. E. Scharff (Eds.), *Fairbairn and the Object Relations Tradition*. London: Karnac, pp. 295–308.

Clarke, G. S. and Scharff, D. E. (2014). *Fairbairn and the Object Relations Tradition*. London: Karnac.

Domenjo, B. A. (2000). Thoughts on the influence of Brentano and Comte on Freud's work. *Psychoanalysis and History*, 2(1): 110–118.

Fairbairn, W. R. D. (1944). Endopsychic structure considered in terms of object-relationships. *International Journal of Psycho-Analysis*, 25: 70–92. [Reprinted in Fairbairn (1952), *Psychoanalytic Studies of the Personality*. London & New York: Routledge, 1992, pp. 82–136.]

Fairbairn, W. R. D. (1952). *Psychoanalytic Studies of the Personality*. London and New York: Routledge, 1992.

Ferenczi, S. (1933). Confusion of the tongues between the adults and the child – (The language of tenderness and of passion). *International Journal of Psycho-Analysis*, 1949, 30: 225–230. Also in *Contemporary Psychoanalysis*, 1988, 24: 196–206.

Ferenczi, S. (1985). The clinical diary of Sándor Ferenczi (J. Dupont, Ed., M. Balint and N. Z. Jackson, Trans.). Cambridge, MA: Harvard University Press, 1988. [Originally written in 1932 and first published in French as "*Journal Clinique (janvier–octobre 1932*"), Paris: Payot.]

Foulkes, S. H. (1948). *Introduction to Group-Analytic Psychotherapy: Studies in the Social Interaction of Individuals and Groups*. London: Karnac, 1984. [Original publication, London: Heinemann.]

Foulkes, S. H. (1964). *Therapeutic Group Analysis*. London: Karnac, 1984. [Original publication, London: Allen & Unwin.]

Foulkes, S. H. (1975). *Group-Analytic Psychotherapy: Method and Principles*. London: Gordon & Breach. [Reprinted, London: Karnac, 2012.]

Freud, S. (1900a). *The Interpretation of Dreams. S.E.*, Vol. 4–5. London: Hogarth Mifflin.

Freud, S. (1915c). *Instincts and Their Vicissitudes. S.E.*, Vol. 14. London: Hogarth Mifflin, pp. 109–140.

Freud, S. (1915–16). *Introductory Lectures to Psycho-Analysis – Parts I and 2, S.E.*, Vol. 22. London: Hogarth Mifflin, pp. 1–182.

Freud, S. (1930a). *Civilization and its Discontents. S.E.*, Vol. 21. London: Hogarth Mifflin, pp. 64–145.

Freud, S. (1933a). *New Introductory Lectures to Psycho-Analysis, S.E.*, Vol. 22. London: Hogarth Mifflin, pp. 1–182.

Freud, S. (1950a). *Project for a Scientific Psychology. S.E.*, Vol. 1. London: Hogarth Mifflin. [Written in 1885.], pp. 281–391.

Freud, S. and Breuer, J. (1895d). *Studies on Hysteria. S.E.*, Vol. 2. London: Hogarth Mifflin.

Goldman, D. (1993). *In Search of the Real: The Origins and Originality of D. W. Winnicott*. Northvale, NJ & London: Aronson.

Greenberg, J. R. and Mitchell, S. A. (1983). *Object Relations in Psychoanalytic Theory*. Cambridge, MA: Harvard University Press.

Guntrip, H. (1961). *Personality Structure and Human Interaction: The Developing Synthesis of Psychodynamic Theory*. London: Hogarth Mifflin. [Reprinted, London, Karnac, 2011.]

Guntrip, H. (1975). My experience of analysis with Fairbairn and Winnicott – (How complete a result does psycho-analytic therapy achieve?). *International Review of Psycho-Analysis*, 2: 145–156. [Reprinted, *International Journal of Psycho-Analysis*, 77: 739–754.]

Hernández Hernández, R. (2010). Inconsciente y concepción del mundo [The unconscious and the *Weltanschauung*]. Unpublished Doctor in Psychotherapy Dissertation, Centre for Graduate Studies, Mexican Psychoanalytic Association, Mexico City.

Hernández-Tubert, R. (2000). El principio de exclusión en el desarrollo del movimiento psicoanalítico [The principle of exclusion in the development of the psychoanalytical movement]. Read at the 8th International Meeting of the International Association for the History of Psychoanalysis, Versailles, France, June.

Hernández-Tubert, R. (2009). Inconsciente y concepción del mundo. Implicaciones filosóficas y psicoanalíticas [The unconscious and the *Weltanschauung*: Philosophical and psychoanalytical implications]. In R. Blanco Beledo (Ed.), *Filosofía ¿y? Psicoanálisis* [Philosophy and (?) psychoanalysis]. Mexico City: Universidad Nacional Autónoma de México, Centro de Investigaciones Interdisciplinarias en Ciencias y Humanidades, pp. 79–104.

Hernández-Tubert, R. (2011). Hacia un nuevo paradigma del ser humano: la confluencia del psicoanálisis y la hermenéutica analógica [Toward a new paradigm of the human being: The confluence of psychoanalysis and analogical hermeneutics]. Read in the 47th International Psychoanalytical Congress Mexico City, August.

Hernández-Tubert. (2015). Inclusion and exclusion in psychoanalysis: From splitting to integration in our theory and practice. *Canadian Journal of Psychoanalysis*, 23(1): 179–186.

Kohon, G. (Ed.) (1986). *The British School of Psychoanalysis: The Independent Tradition*. London: Free Association Books.

Losso, R., Setton, L. S. de and Scharff, D. E. (Eds.) (2017). *The Linked Self in Psychoanalysis: The Pioneering Work of Enrique Pichon Riviere*. London: Karnac.

Masson, J. M. (1985). *The Complete Letters of Sigmund Freud to Wilhelm Fliess, 1887–1904*. Cambridge, MA: The Belknap Press of Harvard University Press.

Pichon-Rivière, E. (1971a). *El proceso grupal. Del psicoanálisis a la psicología social (1)* [The group process: From psychoanalysis to social psychology (1)]. Buenos Aires: Nueva Visión.

Pichon-Rivière, E. (1979). *Teoría del vínculo* [Theory of the link]. Buenos Aires: Nueva Visión.

Rodman, F. (1987). Introduction. In Winnicott (1987), F. R. Rodman (Ed.), *The Spontaneous Gesture: Selected Letters of D. W. Winnicott*. Cambridge, MA: Harvard University, pp. xiii–xxxiii.

Rudnytsky, P. (2000). *Psychoanalytic Conversation: Interviews with Clinicians, Commentators, and Critics*. Hillsdale, NJ: Academic Press.

Stern, D. B. (2013a). Field theory in psychoanalysis, Part I: Harry Stack Sullivan and Madeleine and Willy Baranger. *Psychoanalytic Dialogues*, 23: 487–501.

Stern, D. B. (2013b). Field theory in psychoanalysis, part 2: Bionian field theory and contemporary interpersonal/relational psychoanalysis. *Psychoanalytic Dialogues*, 23: 630–645.

Tubert-Oklander, J. (2007). The whole and the parts: Working in the analytic field. *Psychoanalytic Dialogues*, 17(1): 115–132.

Tubert-Oklander, J. (2008). Las contradicciones de Freud y el carácter híbrido del psicoanálisis [Freud's contradictions and the hybrid character of psychoanalysis]. In J. Tubert-Oklander. and M. Beuchot Puente (Eds.), *Ciencia mestiza. Psicoanálisis y hermenéutica analógica* [Hybrid science: Psychoanalysis and analogical hermeneutics]. Mexico City: Torres, pp. 50–72.

Tubert-Oklander, J. (2014a). *The One and the Many: Relational Psychoanalysis and Group Analysis*. London: Karnac.

Tubert-Oklander, J. (2014b), The icon and the idol: The place of Freud and other founding fathers and mothers in psychoanalytic identity and education. In J. Tubert-Oklander (Ed.), *The One and the Many: Relational Psychoanalysis and Group Analysis*, 1994. London: Karnac, pp. 113–156.

Tubert-Oklander, J. (2014c). A Hermes in London: The subtlety of interpretation in Donald Winnicott's clinic. In J. Tubert-Oklander (Ed.), *The One and the Many: Relational Psychoanalysis and Group Analysis, 1994*. London: Karnac, pp. 157–179.

Tubert-Oklander, J. (2016). The quest for the real. In G. Legorreta and L. J. Brown (Eds.), *On Freud's "Formulations on the Two Principles of Mental Functioning"*. London: Karnac.

Tubert-Oklander, J. (2017a). Psychoanalysis and group analysis: Toward a new paradigm of the human being. Read at the Psychoanalytic Institute of Northern California, San Francisco,

January 3, 2017. Published electronically in the blog Juan Tubert-Oklander (English). Retrieved from http://tubert-oklander-english.blogspot.mx/2017/02/psychoanalysis-and-group-analysis.html

Tubert-Oklander, J. (2017b). Field theories and process theories. In M. Katz, R. Cassorla. and G. Civitarese (Eds.), *Advances in Contemporary Psychoanalytic Field Theory: Concept and Future Development*. London & New York: Routledge.

Tubert-Oklander, J. (2017c). Donald Winnicott: Un revolucionario a pesar suyo [Donald Winnicott: A revolutionary in spite of himself]. Read at the 16th Latin-American Conference in the Thought of D. Winnicott. Mexico City, November 2017. Published electronically in the blog Juan Tubert-Oklander (Español). Retrieved from http://jtubertoklander.blogspot.com/2017/12/donald-winnicott-un-revolucionario.html

Tubert-Oklander, J. (2018). Is Fairbairn still at large? *Contemporary Psychoanalysis*, 54(1): 201–228.

Tubert-Oklander, J. (2019). Beyond psychoanalysis and group analysis: The urgent need for a new paradigm of the human being. 43rd S. H. Foulkes Annual lecture. London: Group-Analytic Society International, May 2019.

Tubert-Oklander, J. and Hernández de Tubert, R. (2004). *Operative Groups: The Latin-American Approach to Group Analysis*. London: Jessica Kingsley.

Winnicott, D. W. (1955). Metapsychological and clinical aspects of regression within the psycho-analytical set-up. *International Journal of Psycho-Analysis*, 36: 16–26. [Reprinted in (1958–1975), *Through Paediatrics to Psycho-Analysis*, Second Edition. London: Hogarth Mifflin, pp. 278–294.]

Winnicott, D. W. (1956). Letter to W. Clifford M. Scott, 26 December. Quoted by Brett Kahr in *D. W. Winnicott: A Biographical Portrait*. London: Karnac, 1996, p. 70.

Winnicott, D. W. (1958). The capacity to be alone. *International Journal of Psycho-Analysis*, 39: 416–420. [Reprinted in Winnicott (1965), *The Maturational Processes and the Facilitating Environment: Studies in the Theory of Emotional Development*. London: Hogarth Mifflin, pp. 29–36.]

Winnicott, D. W. (1960). Ego distortion in terms of a true and false self. In D. W. Winnicott (Ed.), *The Maturational Processes and the Facilitating Environment: Studies in the Theory of Emotional Development*, 1965. London: Hogarth Mifflin, pp. 140–152.

Winnicott, D. W. (1962). A personal view of the Kleinian contribution. In D. W. Winnicott (Ed.), *The Maturational Processes and the Facilitating Environment: Studies in the Theory of Emotional Development*, 1965. London: Hogarth Mifflin, pp. 171–178.

Winnicott, D. W. (1963). From dependence toward independence in the development of the individual. In D. W. Winnicott (Ed.), *The Maturational Processes and the Facilitating Environment: Studies in the Theory of Emotional Development*, 1965. London: Hogarth Mifflin, pp. 83–92.

Winnicott, D. W. (1969). The use of an object. *International Journal of Psycho-Analysis*, 50: 711–716. [Reprinted as "The use of an object and relating through identifications" in Winnicott (1971), *Playing and Reality*. London: Tavistock. pp. 86–94.]

Winnicott, D. W. and Khan, M. M. R. (1953). Review of *Psychoanalytic Studies of the Personality*. *International Journal of Psycho-Analysis*, 34: 329–333 [Reprinted in D. W. Winnicott, *Psycho-Analytic Explorations* (pp. 413–422). London: Karnac, 1989.]

8 The use of the object

Personal and clinical reflections

Jill Savege Scharff

"The use of the object" is the theme selected for this book, to which the editor, my husband, David E. Scharff, has invited me to contribute, and so I must write something that fits the theme. What exactly is he looking for? What is an object anyway? In our work as therapists, the term "object" may refer to a literal object, a thing that is used in various ways and that we then interpret as a metaphor for a mental function. Perhaps that would be interesting to write about. "Object" may refer to the external object, a term for an actual person such as a significant other. I always think that expression is a bit weird and could be boring. More interesting, "object" may refer to the internal object, a structure in the mind that is a trace of interactions with and experience of a significant other in the formative years. Then again, "object" is often used as shorthand for "internal object relationship" and thus has a more complex meaning, referring to both an internal object and the part of the ego that relates to it and all the affects that connect them (Scharff and Scharff, 2005). So which of these should I write about?

Frankly facing the task of beginning to write this chapter was not easy. I couldn't decide. I couldn't settle. I felt stuck. So, I tried to go to sleep. I was hoping that as I slept, my unconscious would give me the answer or, better yet, write the chapter for me. But my unconscious said, "No way. But I will give you a dream, so at least you can sleep."

The dream as an object

In my dream, I saw David indoors in a corridor in January, wearing a suit made of patches of cotton fabric in a green, blue and purple Madras pattern and a bow-tie. I thought it looked fine, but the fabric was unexpectedly lightweight for winter. A woman told him his suit was ridiculous. He ignored her, but I knew he was irritated. When she persisted in criticizing him, he said, "Enough. Meet me downstairs. We need to have a text meeting." I was glad he confronted her, but I was giggling to myself that the phrase is text message not text meeting, and he seemed ridiculous using such an odd description for a meeting.

In this dream, the patchwork of David's suit reminds me of a favorite pair of patchwork tie-dyed pants I had in Scotland before I knew him and also of an American version of a Scottish plaid, but the colors of the suit are the colors of the marketing materials for the International Psychotherapy Institute (IPI), which we founded. The corridor setting reminds me of the Rockville conference hotel where we hold in-residence training courses. The light weight of his suit makes me think of April, when graduation occurs. The woman who was angry at David looks like a patient of mine who has been angry at her husband and critical of his way of doing things, while she does nothing but now is afraid of losing him. The word "text" seems to refer to the missing text of this chapter that I owe him but that is not yet written. He hasn't confronted me about getting the chapter written in time but he has been teasing me about how ridiculous it is that I will do everything else first – clean my desk, arrange family dinners, clean up all the administrative tasks that must be done – before I will write. And is there a message in the dream about my chapter?

The dream as an anxiety release object did let me sleep, and I did wake up with the dream as an object for contemplation and a start for my essay. It shows me that David is being patient while controlling his irritation with me, that I rebel against the task, and that I would rather ridicule David than co-operate. I would rather ridicule him than feel so ridiculous and inept myself. I would rather it were April, after the Master Speakers date, so that I could be watching students graduate rather than step up myself. I have to agree with my dream that indeed it is time for a text meeting. I have to stop my use of the term "object" as a verb to mean "I object" and start creating a chapter, thanks to the work done in the dream. The dream has given the format to "suit" the theme of the book. The book will be a patchwork of chapters, each of them an association to "the object." My chapter will be one of the patches. And within my chapter will be many smaller patches comprising my many associations to the term "the object."

Now I can look back on the dream itself as an object. It is an object for anxiety discharge, for contemplation of the unconscious roots of resistance, for taking back unconscious projective identifications and freeing the ego for work.

The literal object: use of the computer as an object

With the advent of technology, we have ready access to computers and hand-held devices for computation, text messaging, audiovisual communication, memory storage, and games. These are objects that can enhance our capabilities and expose our deficiencies as they challenge us beyond our expertise. Children are growing up with technology as part of their environment, and they relate to technical devices intuitively. To them the devices are familiar extensions of themselves and the world around them. Using Pichon-Rivière's link theory (Losso, Setton and Scharff, 2017), we might say that these technology objects are part of the link into which these people are born and upon which they will exert an impact as they use them in more and various ways that we cannot yet imagine. These objects are also exciting and frustrating in offering immense possibilities and then leaving you in the lurch as the screen goes dark, the Internet connection is lost, or malware corrupts the system. Email can become a persecuting object driving a relentless pace of interaction and creating a record that can come back to haunt you.

For some patients who live remote from a major center, technology-assisted treatment and supervision have been a lifeline, a sustaining object. For analysts who accept these patients, teleanalysis has been a secret, a guilt-ridden object that can draw attack and shaming (Scharff, 2013, 2015, 2017, 2018). According to conservative, traditional analysts, "This is not analysis!" But teleanalysis has a specific setting, a frame of treatment, a private space for reflection, a focus on the unconscious, and in that setting the analytic process occurs through transference and countertransference and the ensuing interpretation leads to therapeutic action. But the bodies are not in the same room, there is no bodily communication, and some people say that therefore there cannot be an analytic process because it is not real. So, for a clinician who does accept patients from afar, teleanalysis has become a controversial object about which study and research may bring validation of its worth.

During distance analysis or therapy of individuals or couples, the technology itself becomes an object of study too. Just as the traditional analyst works with displacement of unconscious desire onto objects outside the transference, the teleanalyst notes that the transference is displaced to the computer screen, the bandwidth, and the choice of setting and gathers it from there to himself. Failure to arrange for adequate bandwidth may be a way of expressing resistance to treatment. It is tempting for the technology novice, the "digital immigrant," to brush past technical problems so as to avoid noticing anxiety about the use of the technology and ineptness with equipment. The teleanalyst is vulnerable to viewing technology as a shaming object and wants to deny its power. But to erase the impact of a failed connection is to miss the opportunity to respond to it as an empathic failure, a sudden deletion of the connection between the preceding thought, feeling, or interaction. When teletherapy is a trusted object, we can proceed to interpret the abandonment anxiety of the failed connection – and that may take us to a discussion of its connection to the maternal void and ultimately to issues of life and death.

The use of the body as an object

The body as a quantified object

How many of my women friends and colleagues use smart watches or Fitbits to track the biological functioning of their own bodies and of their babies! This gives them a feeling of control over sleep and dreaming, exercise (10,000 steps a day!), heart rhythm, and breathing rate and over the baby's input and output, its sleep and wake cycles. I have heard this described as the quantified self (Wolf, 2009), but I think of it as the quantified object. The body becomes an object of the mind rather than the spontaneous source of sensation that drives the formation of the self.

The use of the female body as an object

It's all over the news that women have been putting up for years with sexual aggression and attacks on their competence at work by being reduced to sexual objects. We have been scared of getting physically hurt, accused of being provocative, and left with ruined reputations, too scared to speak up and accuse the perpetrator on whom we are dependent for income and promotion. We are afraid that blame will be turned on us. In non-violent situations, there is discomfort, if not fear. As a young psychiatrist I was viewed as fair game by a senior psychiatrist I worked for. This is a man of integrity who would never have cheated on his wife, but he saw no reason not to comment on my figure. He would loudly propose taking me into the bushes. There was no inappropriate touching. I was not afraid that there might be because I knew he did not mean it, but it was excruciatingly embarrassing to me because I had no idea how to handle it, and so it kept happening. What kind of object was he to me? A man who could break through my defense of being a serious MD to make everyone around see me as a woman to flirt with, a woman who was dependent on him for a job and a performance review, a young woman who didn't know how to play that game and felt pathetically in need of a champion. When a woman is used as an object, she finds it very difficult to be herself and to speak to the issue in a way that does not then treat the man as an object. When we speak about the use of the object, we are really talking about the failure to use the self effectively.

Pregnant women are exposed to lots of non-consensual touching. I am not talking about those times when a woman invites a friend or family member to feel the baby move. I am talking about those times when strangers feel entitled to pat the swollen belly. Some indulge in telling the woman horror stories from their deliveries, and others talk about damaged babies. As a pregnant psychiatrist, I was in class at an analytic institute where most of the teachers were MDs. When one of the teachers saw that I was pregnant, he said that he would have to start carrying his penknife around with him in case he had to do a quick C-section. Clearly the pregnant belly, associated as it is with intercourse, is an object of fascination and the growing fetus an object of envy as well as of hope and wonder. On that occasion I felt a lot of unconscious aggression in my teacher's medical bravado.

As a child and family therapist, I note the way that my body is used as an object. In family therapy, as part of a game, a young boy taped my mouth shut with electrical tape, blindfolded me with a piece of cloth, and spun me around in my office chair so that I could not see what was happening or locate myself in relation to the family, and therefore I could not speak to the dynamics. Of course, I could imagine the family, I know my office well, and I could speak past the tape. I said that he wanted me to know how it felt to be in that family. It must feel so unsafe to look and see what is happening and speak about it that he could feel like he was being spun around by all the forces in the family, all the more in the session with me because our task was to explore the family situation and try to understand it together. His use of me as an object gave me access to his self-experience of his family.

The unpossessible object

The unpossessible object for the needy child

In the autistic child, a child whose emotional and cognitive deficits lead to an inner feeling of spacelessness and mindlessness, the autistic self is dismantled into its sensual components that attach themselves to the most stimulating object of the moment (Meltzer, 2008). This gives a vacuous feeling of omnipotent control over and separation from its objects but leaves the child's mind with a feeling of falling into bits. This feeling of the dismantling of the self leads to extreme dependence on the mental functions of an external object, and not just on the care, holding and handling provided. Because of the unfortunate combination of the inadequacy of the child's equipment and the mother's limitations, a fundamental failure of dependence occurs. The child comes into therapy or analysis and, again, the container-as-object, now in the form of the therapist, is experienced as totally untrustworthy and must be held in place or entered as a way of taking control of it by a kind of fusion rather than inter-relating. This fusion with the object is seen in behavior such as burrowing into the therapist, using the therapist's hands to accomplish manipulations, and demanding to use the therapist's body as if it were furniture. In such cases the therapist may usefully allow a "degree of permissiveness with regard to physical contact, in touching, looking, smelling and tasting." The children are intrusive, highly sensual, and possessive, as if they were desperately trying to possess an unpossessible object by adhering to and capturing its surface qualities but sadly finding it permanently devoid of substance.

The unpossessible object for the unrequited lover

Another variety of unpossessible object is seen in the situation of an adult woman who longs for a lost lover. What or who does he represent to her? What has she projected into her attachment to him? One such woman is Lilia, whose longing is extreme and keeps her frozen in place as a single woman.

Lilia makes a small salary, is an excellent money manager, and is able to pay me a reasonable reduced fee for once-a-week therapy. She is not able to pay for more in terms of time or money. She is a good patient, walking at least 30 minutes to my office, always on time. She is quite depressed and slow to get around to her own problems and begins most sessions with a passionate statement about her latest blog on democratic political ideals, especially gun control, global responsibility, diversity, and social service. She works in the non-profit world and wears simple clothes and no makeup, her short blond hair swept behind her ears. I often feel I would like to fix her to bring out her beauty, and I recognize in that a mother's wish to have her daughter look attractive.

Lilia's presenting symptom is that she cannot get over the pain of losing a man with whom she had a wonderful intimate relationship for less than a year, now six years ago. His name was Pablo, and he came from Panama, so his English was excellent. They met in Kazakhstan, where each of them was doing service abroad. She thought at first that this would be just a fling lasting a couple of months before their posting ended, but it became a wonderful, warm relationship, and Pablo visited the United States and stayed with her and her family. Then he got a job in a remote part of South America, and he expected her to emigrate to be with him. But she didn't speak Spanish and didn't have a work permit, and, although she wanted to be with him right away, she decided to wait, took a job in New York, and informed him that she couldn't join him yet. She expected to continue the relationship on a commuting basis, but he took her decision as a rejection. He didn't come to the United States, and he didn't fight for her to come to the country where he was then living or ease her way there. Lilia looks back on her decision as a response to some problems in the relationship that she hadn't acknowledged, his way of making assumptions about her relationship to him without discussion of her fears and needs, and also her fear of the unknown. But that insight didn't reconcile her to her situation.

Lilia constantly tortures herself with thoughts of how her life might have been different had she gone to be with Pablo. Since communication was so difficult, she went to South America to see him in person and hoped to work it out. That was five years ago. She said, "He was glad to see me, we went out and had fun but he was treating me like an old friend, and there were always these two other women with us. He said I had changed. I was too afraid to ask him how I had changed, and I just acted badly, crying, and jealous and screaming about feeling excluded. No way to get someone back. He said he was 'done with it.' And I am still crying about it years later. So, a couple months ago I went again to see him to settle it once and for all. There was so little likelihood it could work, but I had to try it. And again, he was pleased to see me, we had fun, and again, he was with someone else. I am glad I didn't act badly, but I am still so torn up about it."

Both times she has been faced with the reality of Pablo's current attachment to another woman and of his interest in her purely as a friend. She seemed to me to be in an Oedipal loser situation and to be behaving out of control, which is an aspect of her father that she can't stand and fears. Yet the lost love is still firmly installed as a desired and frustrating love object in her heart and mind. When I described the *hold* she let him have on her, Lilia thought I said *hole*. This helped me see the defensive reason for her installing him as an internal object to fill a hole and to keep her from risking involvement with any other man, but I didn't yet know the reason.

In the session before the one I will present, Lilia explained, "I had always chosen where to live and work on the basis of a sense of calling. This was the first time *I thought with my head, not my heart*, and I have been regretting it ever since. I was ready to go on a tourist visa, but I was afraid. I need an internal process to figure out the right decision, and he didn't give me that. *I was thinking with my heart not my head*, and something was telling me don't go. He was slow to respond on G-chat. Instead of confronting him and saying I feel you are not fully engaged, not helping me with this transition, I just shut down, and moved to DC for a safe job." I noted the reversal of heart and head but waited to see what I could make of it.

In the next session, she began by telling me she had noticed two things about herself: "I really want you to like me so that I will get what I need from therapy and get better, *and* I am trying not to cry, which could make you think that I am just like those dramatic people you always hear talking about their parents in therapy on television." I had noticed she was leaning forward talking and gesticulating and smiling as if to engage me actively because she was unable to assume

I would listen and keep my commitment. She often tells me successful things she has done at work activity to make me admire her and delay work on her insecurities. I also noted that she does cry by the end of sessions, which feels like a relief to me, not a dramatic maneuver at all. I want her to cry or not cry, just be herself as we try to get at her underlying problems.

Lilia said, "My Dad is the most introverted person you will ever meet, and I love it that he doesn't give a crap about what people expect of him in the Hamptons where they live. But at home I hate it that he is like a terrorist suddenly getting so angry and being impossible. And my mother can't protect us from it. On the other hand, he is really there. He spent all his money on education for us and adventure vacations. And our college tuition was fully funded. Even though he had a stroke, we had no worries about staying in school. I drove down from school to see him every week for eight weeks when he was recovering. I am so glad I did that."

I asked about the illness, and she began to cry.

"Yeah he had a stroke. I was in shock. I called my sister and asked her what we would do if he didn't survive. She just said calmly she would take Mom to live with her, and Mom could take care of the grandchildren. Maybe it would be better for Mom, but that is the way my sister is. She deals. But then he had a good response to rehab, and he can still work full-time.

"After the stroke he dropped from 350 pounds to 250. But that is still too heavy for his height. I told him I couldn't fight him on it anymore. If he wants be fat and drop dead of another stroke or a heart attack, he will just have to do it." Lilia is crying again. "My Mom never said anything about his weight. She doesn't fight about anything at all. Well, my Mom just isn't there. Call her up for a conversation and she talks about the news and the weather. I never learn anything about her, or who she is apart from him."

I said, "Your sister responded to the threat of losing your father in terms of your mother's needs. But what about the effect on *you* of losing your Dad? Then you would be left with only your mother."

Lilia started to cry again.

I said, "How does all this connect to you?"

She asked, "What do you mean?"

I said, "Well, your mother is subsumed in your father. He is big and she is tiny. You feel she is nothing for you to relate to."

"Yes, she is all about him. I just don't know who she is. I wish she had a passion, but she doesn't. She just gets consumed in him. Oh, she took a class in botany, which could be a great thing, but it was just to pass the time. I can relate to that, though. Sometimes I just want the time to pass so I can go to sleep and the pain will stop. I hurt all the time. The first time I felt it was in seventh grade when the girls suddenly excluded me from the clique."

I asked if she has an image of the pain.

She said, "I feel that there is pipe stuck through my heart, and my heart is beating around it."

I remembered her references in the previous session to thinking with her heart or her head. I said again, "Let's see how this connects to you. You are like your father in being education oriented, ambitious, and passionate about education, human rights, and women's issues. But you are like your mother in being subsumed in Pablo. You both make the man into a wonderful, powerful object for you to desire and feel hurt by. Pablo is so big in your life, and he just sits there in your heart, and you are not able to think of making room for any other man to make a relationship with. We can't know why your mother lives through your father, but we can see that you use Pablo like a pipe to fill the hole that's left in your heart from before you ever met him."

It seems that Lilia's identification with her mother's way of using her husband as an object in which to lose herself drove the fantasy of immersing herself in life with Pablo in his culture, but because of actual lack of connection to her mother's self she reacted against that identification and decided not to go. Now it seems that Lilia's fighting for Pablo is a way of creating a man to make up for what is missing in her relationship with her mother and an experience of losing out to another woman, as the child must lose out to her mother who is already her father's wife. Is Lilia's fight for Pablo also a way of exploring whether her father's angry outbursts are not simply a response to stress, as claimed, but rather a reaction to her mother's emotional absence and a search for a present but unpossessible object?

The patient as the therapist's object

The valued and envied object

At this point in my career, most of my adult patients are mental health professionals. I feel an ethical responsibility to restrict my use of their material for teaching purposes. So, although in the office context these patients are gifted in their capacity for deep unconscious communication and analysis, in the teaching setting they are off limits. These are people who respond well to analysis, who engage with me, fight with me, and make reparation to me and in whose sessions I generally feel that I am a good analyst. Of course, you will have to take my word for it. You might not agree at all. But I still have the fantasy that if I presented their sessions, they would make me look good. So what kind of an object is such a patient? A narcissistically gratifying object, a precious hidden gem, but one that leaves me depleted of the opportunity for external validation – or course correction – from helpful colleagues, which leaves me and them vulnerable to countertransference mistakes, to overvaluation, and to living through them. Some patients make you feel like a talented analyst when others do not. I am reminded of Winnicott's compliment to Guntrip as the patient who made him look good whereas the chap before him did not (Guntrip, 1975, p. 153). So, these patients are reassuring objects to me. And yet if they are candidates in training, the institutional context bears down on the analysis, and these treasured objects are exposed to attack that may have more to do with the institution's envy of the analyst for having such a candidate to work with than anything to do with the candidate himself. Here the candidate is an object for displaced attack.

The elusive object

In my case, the patient who does not make me look good is the one I could more easily present, the one who showed up in my dream. But I find I don't want to. She is an at-home mother who does substitute elementary school teaching. So, she has a late-afternoon appointment time, which is when I am most tired. She is intelligent, pretty, and devoted to her family. She is a good patient, punctual, reliable, flexible, and compliant. She talks freely about her life, and her feelings of rejection by her husband, who does not join her interest in social life and tennis, and her child, who is secretive about her activities and her feelings. She is open about her depression and negativity, her jealousy of people with confidence, and her total lack of confidence in her ability despite positive feedback at work. She brings in notes on her dreams, which are so long and complicated that she cannot remember them, and if I don't write them down, I can't reconstruct them in my mind either. She is not boring, but she is somewhat opaque to me. She is afraid that no matter how hard she tries or how faithfully she attends, she will never get to the root of her lack of confidence.

As I work with this patient, I feel I am not getting beyond the surface. She does not engage with me as the others do. I make interpretations and she often accepts them and elaborates on them, but they don't seem to make a difference. She still feels that she is not the woman she wants to be. She has many friends, never more in evidence than now when her daughter is ill, but she feels unworthy of their care and basically does not feel loved. It feels as if my therapeutic love is not enough either. Her resistance is shown not against the frame or in direct challenges to me but against herself and me as the person with therapeutic ambitions. Perhaps she doesn't want me to feel better about myself than she does. This patient is a test of analysis and of me as her analyst. In this case the patient is an elusive object.

The ideal object, the denigrated therapist

My first male analytic patient was an ideal object to me. I was enchanted by his discourse, fascinated by his accent, and impressed by his access to Washington political life. I overlooked that fact that he made no money, that he paid me from his inheritance less than I paid my supervisor, and that his denigration of his wife and neglect of his children would soon fall upon me. My supervisor was equally enchanted with the patient and with me. He listened intently, never interrupted, and at the end of the session murmured something approving. After the patient had been in analysis for two years, I got pregnant. The supervisor instructed me to make no announcement, to wait until it appeared in the man's associations. But the man ignored my pregnancy, preferring to think that I was getting fat. This man was an only child and had never had to deal with a rival for his mother's devotion. When his children were born, he hated his wife being so preoccupied with them. When my imminent delivery could be avoided no longer, he apparently accepted that I would be away on maternity leave and return in two months. But, a week after delivery, he called up my husband to ask him what I had had, a boy or a girl. David told him that mother and baby are both well and any other questions he might take up with me on my return. The man was furious. He returned after the two months, deeply offended at my husband's reply. He said, "I called to express my concern for you, but your husband was rude, like an officious clerk at a ticket counter saying next counter please." I was sympathetic to his feeling of rejection and appreciative of his concern. But when I too did not answer his question, he quit, and he did not answer my letters asking for closure. He did not pay the balance of my bill, left unpaid for two months before my maternity leave began, and I had to write it off. I had abandoned him for a husband and a baby, and we had denied him access to knowledge about our baby. Mutual idealization defaulted to denigration and traumatic loss. This overvalued first patient became a disappointing object because I had disappointed him in failing to accept his concern and, I might add, in failing to see what a baby he was in real-life and what a baby I was in doing my first analysis.

The reparative object

More recently I had a similarly narcissistic male patient. His intellect was quite amazing, but thanks to my earlier experience I was not bewitched. I could be appreciative, but also call him on the narcissism of his intellectual defense and help him heal himself. Unlike my first case, he became a reparative object for me.

The memorable object

Another woman patient was directly challenging to me. She was furious at me much of the time because she felt that I was refusing to agree to her demands that I love her. She had lost her mother in a traumatic way and really felt the need of maternal care. On the couch, what she needed to do was to scream at me in rage at all she had lost so that she could stop being so vicious with people in her life. Sometimes I hated her as much as she hated me. She and I had lengthy engagement in dark hours, affect storms, and hurts until her neurosis, and its installation in the transference/countertransference dynamic, was represented in a dream as a point on the shore that became smaller and smaller as she was rowing out away from it. At the end of her successful analysis she told me that she realized that what she had had from me was not love as such but love such as it is. And it had been what she needed. This was years ago during my training, but her conclusion about love has remained with me, and so has she. She is a highly valued object in my internal world as an analyst, rather like a first love, let go of, grown beyond, but never forgotten.

Summary

In this chapter I explored the meaning of the term "the object." I addressed the literal object, such as the computer used as an object for interpretive work in teleanalysis. I look at the use of the body as an object – especially the female body, very topical and always strikingly relevant for the child therapist. I have illustrated the use of the object in intimate and therapeutic relationships to express, hide, deny, attack, or cohere parts of the self and to absorb desire or hatred. The concluding section featured the patient as the therapist's object.

References

Guntrip, H. (1975). My experience of analysis with Fairbairn and Winnicott. *International Journal of Psycho-Analysis*, 16: 145–156.

Losso, R., Setton, L. and Scharff, D. (2017). *The Linked Self in Psychoanalysis: The Pioneering Work of Enrique Pichon-Rivière*. London: Karnac.

Meltzer, D. (Ed.) (2008). *Explorations in Autism*. London: Karnac.

Scharff, J. (Ed.) (2013). *Psychoanalysis Online: Mental Health, Teletherapy and Training*. London: Karnac.

Scharff, J. (Ed.) (2015). *Psychoanalysis Online 2: Impact of Technology on Development, Training and Therapy*. London: Karnac.

Scharff, J. (Ed.) (2017). *Psychoanalysis Online 3: The Teleanalytic Setting*. London: Karnac.

Scharff, J. (Ed.) (2018). *Psychoanalysis Online 4: Teleanalytic Practice, Clinical Research and Teaching*. London: Karnac.

Scharff, J. S. and Scharff, D. E. (2005). *The Primer of Object Relations*, 2nd Edition. Lanham, MD: Jason Aronson.

Wolf, G. (2009). Know thyself: Tracking every facet of life; from sleep to mood to pain. *Wired Magazine*, 24(7): 365.

Epilogue

David E. Scharff

The idea of how we use others has spawned diverse theories, from the intersubjective way that we co-create experience with others to the theorists of the link in South America who see the encounter with others as always constituting a challenge to the continuity of our psychic selves.

In this volume, written largely from the vantage of psychoanalytic object relations, the contributors have looked at how we encounter, use, and relate to others from a number of perspectives. Listening to and, later, reading the thinking of each contributor has expanded my own way of seeing the psychoanalytic object. The objects we encounter as the history of each patient comes to life through daily analytic work show us details about our patients as their objects acquire ever more vivid qualities, brought into focus as we probe the depths of our patients' unconscious. As we do so, we also come to constitute an increasingly complex object for each patient.

In this process, we are gradually transformed from seeming to them to be a new edition of old objects to becoming an object of a new kind. In this way we hope to disrupt how they have seen and related to their old objects. We hope to foster growth by being developmental objects, we offer to be transference objects, and ultimately, we aspire to become transformational objects.

In this way, we lend ourselves to be used in the way Winnicott proposed more than 50 years ago. In his terms, we offer to move from being objects to whom our patients relate, to being there for object use, as patients explore the world of others and move beyond the constraints that bound them when they first sought our help.

I hope that this book, too, will have become an object for use – a guide offering an opportunity to think anew about common clinical dilemmas and, at opportune times, an object that creatively disrupts ways of thinking in order to lead us toward opportunities for growth in our capacity to help our patients.

Index

Note: *Italicized* page numbers indicate a figure on the corresponding page.

For Product Safety Concerns and Information please contact our EU representative GPSR@taylorandfrancis.com
Taylor & Francis Verlag GmbH, Kaufingerstraße 24, 80331 München, Germany

www.ingramcontent.com/pod-product-compliance
Ingram Content Group UK Ltd.
Pitfield, Milton Keynes, MK11 3LW, UK
UKHW022314250926
475702UK00046B/774

* 9 7 8 0 3 6 7 1 8 9 1 5 0 *